Welcome To The Ticcer's Guide

This book has been created to provide information to Tourettic people and their families on TS and related conditions. It is intended to help ticcers develop self-acceptance, confidence, self-understanding, and allow people to become aware of various management strategies. This book switches between addressing parents/carers and Tourettic people themselves as this book is intended not only for the person with TS themselves, but for their whole family as well. This is why terms such as "you" (referring to a Tourettic person) or "your child" (referring to parents) are used interchangeably.

This book will cover not only information on Tourette's, but also information on related conditions such as PANDAS/PANS, OCD, and ADHD.

I hope that the information in this book is helpful and that the information provided gives you some lightbulb moments.

I began writing this guide at the age of 16 after years of struggling with severe tics and OCD. I wanted to give something back to the community, and use my experience to help others with the condition. Now, at age 21, I am finally able to put this book out there with the hope that the information included can be useful. This is what I have learnt growing up with TS, and what I wish I had known sooner.

Disclaimer: I am not a medical professional, so none of the information in this book can be taken as medical advice. This is for educational purposes only.

I hope this book gives you confidence, and gives you an idea on how to adjust to life with TS and accept your unique self!

Page Of Contents

Glossary

- **Ableism:** Discriminatory and prejudiced attitudes towards disabled people
- **ADHD**: Attention Deficit Hyperactivity Disorder
- **ASD**: Autism Spectrum Disorder
- **CBIT**: Comprehensive Behavioral Intervention for Tics
- **CBT**: Cognitive Behavioral Therapy
- **ERP**: Exposure and Response Prevention
- **EHCP**: Education Health and Care Plan
- **FND**: Functional Neurological Disorder
- **IgG**: Immunoglobulin G
- **Inflammatory Cytokines**: Markers of inflammation
- **IVIG**: Intravenous Immunoglobulin
- **MSG**: Monosodium Glutamate
- **OCD**: Obsessive Compulsive Disorder
- **PANDAS**: Pediatric Autoimmune Neuropsychiatric Disorder Associated with Streptococcal Infections
- **PANS**: Pediatric Acute Onset Neuropsychiatric Syndrome
- **Premonitory urge**: The uncomfortable urge that comes before a tic
- **SPD**: Sensory Processing Disorder
- **Ticcer**: A person with Tourette Syndrome or tics
- **TS:** Tourette Syndrome

Chapter One

AN INTRODUCTION TO CONDITIONS THAT CAN CAUSE TICS.

Conditions That Cause Tics

Tourette Syndrome is not the only condition that is known to cause tics - many conditions can cause this symptom. In this chapter, we will explore a variety of conditions that can cause tics, starting with Tourette's.

Tourette Syndrome: Probably the most well-known tic-related condition is Tourette Syndrome, or Tourette's for short.

Tourette Syndrome is a neurological condition that usually starts before the age of 18. It is thought to be genetic as it often runs in families. Tourette Syndrome can be diagnosed when a person has at least one vocal tic and two or more motor tics for over a year, with onset before the age of 18 and the symptoms not being caused by another condition or substance.

People with Tourette Syndrome can experience symptoms other than tics too, such as rage attacks, disinhibition, executive dysfunction, and symptoms from common co-occurring conditions such as ADHD and OCD.

Tourette Syndrome and Persistent Tic Disorders are currently thought to affect 1 in 50 people. The tics caused by Tourette Syndrome are organic tics, meaning that they are caused by a physical or structural difference in the brain or nervous system.

Provisional Tic Disorder: This is the term given to someone who has motor and vocal tics for under a year. Once they hit the year mark their diagnosis will be changed to Tourette Syndrome. However, it is important that other potential diagnoses are considered such as FND or PANDAS/PANS.

Chronic Motor Tic Disorder: This is the diagnosis given when a person has only motor tics for more than a year, not caused by another condition.

Chronic Vocal Tic Disorder: This is the diagnosis given when a person has only vocal tics for more than a year, not caused by another condition.

Functional Tics (From Functional Neurological Disorder): Functional tics are different from organic tics in the sense that they are not caused by a structural issue in the brain. It is often described as "the hardware is normal but the software is glitchy". Functional tics are less likely to be suppressible and are less likely to have a physical premonitory urge before the tic. They can happen without warning. The onset of functional tics usually occurs in the teenage years and has a sudden onset - however, PANDAS should also be ruled out whenever there is a sudden onset. People with FND will often experience other symptoms such as episodic or long-term paralysis in certain areas of the body, non-epileptic seizures, and dystonia. All of these symptoms can also occur as part of PANDAS/PANS, so if these symptoms start with an infection and flare whenever the person is sick, alongside OCD or food restriction, then it is probably PANS.

Tourettism: This is a term used to describe a case where someone has symptoms of Tourette Syndrome from another cause. For example, if a person develops tics as a side effect of medication or from carbon monoxide poisoning they don't have Tourette's as they do not meet diagnostic criteria, but they could be referred to as having "Tourettism".

PANDAS and PANS: PANDAS is a condition triggered by group A Streptococcal infections that causes the immune system to attack part of the brain called the basal ganglia. You have to have either tics, OCD, or both, triggered by a Strep infection to be diagnosed with PANDAS. PANS is similar but it is triggered by many infections other than Strep, such as Influenza or Mycoplasma, and can also be triggered by non-infectious factors. You have to have either OCD or food restriction to be diagnosed with PANS, however many people with PANS also have tics.

Conditions That Can Cause Involuntary Movements Which May Be Mistaken For Tourette's and Tic Disorders:

- **Stereotypic Movement Disorder:** A condition characterized by self-stimulatory movements / stereotypic movements.

- **Sydenham's Chorea:** A post-streptococcal disease causing involuntary dance-like movements, hand-wringing, grimacing, slurred speech, a milkmaid's grip, muscle weakness, restlessness, clumsiness, and jerking movements of the arms and body.

- **Epilepsy**: Myoclonic jerks caused by an epileptic seizure may be mistaken for tics. Epileptic seizures do not have the ability to be suppressed and can be detected on an EEG monitor.

A note on "anxiety tics":

Tics are not typically listed as a symptom of anxiety, and "anxiety tics" is not an official diagnostic term. It is very common for tics to get worse with stress and anxiety in people with Tourette's, PANDAS, PANS, and other conditions that can cause tics, but that doesn't mean that anxiety is the cause. This is why so many people with Tourette's and PANDAS/PANS are misdiagnosed as having "anxiety tics", which leads to diagnostic delay and inappropriate symptom management.

When doctors blame tics on anxiety without considering the possibility of Tourette Syndrome, or a similar condition like PANS, this is usually a form of medical gaslighting. Girls are particularly prone to this kind of misdiagnosis due to medical misogyny.

Why Is It Important To Distinguish Between PANDAS/PANS, FND and Tourette Syndrome?

- Despite causing similar symptoms, PANDAS/PANS, FND, and Tourette Syndrome are all managed differently. Due to this, the correct diagnosis is important so that the condition can be managed effectively. PANDAS/PANS is often managed through the use of antimicrobial medications, immunomodulatory interventions, and anti-inflammatory treatments. FND is usually managed by treating the underlying triggers such as anxiety, depression, or PTSD. Tourette Syndrome is conventionally managed through the use of CBIT and medications such as neuroleptics.

- If a person receives an incorrect diagnosis, they may feel confused if new symptoms arise that cannot be attributed to the diagnosis they were given. For example, if a person is diagnosed with Tourette Syndrome but then goes on to contract an infection which triggers psychosis, restrictive eating, and dystonic symptoms - they will likely be extremely confused and concerned. Whereas if a person was correctly diagnosed with PANDAS/PANS then they would have an idea of why that happened and therefore would be less confused. They would also be able to access the appropriate treatment for a flare quicker with a correct diagnosis.

- A person may feel misunderstood within the Tourette's community if they have actually been misdiagnosed and don't really have Tourette's. For example, a person with undiagnosed functional tics may be confused when they hear people in the Tourette's community talking about tic suppression and premonitory urges as they may not experience this. The correct diagnosis may allow the person to connect with others who really understand what they are going through, such as other people with functional tics (tics caused by FND.)

Tics come and go, so if you have a tic that is particularly troublesome then know that it may pass soon and be replaced by a less distressing tic.

Chapter Two

TYPES OF TICS

What Is A Tic?

In this chapter, we are discussing the different types of tics. Tics can present in many different ways, but before we dive into the many different complex ways that tics present, we must answer the question "What is a tic?"

A tic is an involuntary movement or vocalization (and sometimes a thought or sensation.) Tics change over time and can be replaced by other tics. They can wax and wane depending on any triggering factors. Tics can be simple or complex and anything the human body can possibly do could be a tic. A simple motor tic could include nose twitching and a complex motor tic could include running out the door. An example of a simple vocal tic could be throat clearing and a complex vocal tic could include yelling a whole phrase. For some people, a strong sensation (premonitory urge) can come before a tic and can cause immense discomfort. Some people can temporarily hold in their tics for certain periods of time (tic suppression) however this is often harmful for the individual therefore it should be actively discouraged as it can lead to rebounds of extreme tics, rage attacks, migraines, anxiety and other unwanted symptoms later on when in a safe environment.

Tic suppression also causes the premonitory urge to accumulate and therefore can be very distressing and can even hurt for some people. Suppressing tics can sometimes feel like you can't breathe so it can become physically intolerable, this can be like holding your breath.

What Is A Premonitory Urge?

A premonitory urge is a sensation that usually comes before a tic, it can be very uncomfortable and distressing to the person experiencing it. Not everyone with tics experiences the premonitory urge but for some people, it is very prominent, and therefore tic suppression can cause an extreme rebound later on and cause a lot of discomfort as tics and other symptoms that are held in will always have to come out at some time. The urge can occur in any part of the body (and sometimes out of the body - see phantom tics.) The premonitory urge doesn't necessarily occur in the localized area where the tic is present. The sensation feels different for everyone and often different tics have different urges - it could feel like an accumulation of pressure, a balloon in your chest, an itch, something sticking to the skin, something trapped inside of us, a tingling feeling, or just general discomfort. Some people may not be aware of the urge at a young age but may notice it more as they age, but some people are aware of it at a very young age.

Anything can be a tic, but the following list includes some examples:

Simple Vocal Tics: Squeaking, throat clearing, sniffing, tongue clicking, making syllable sounds, gulping, sighing, coughing, grunting.

Simple Motor Tics: Hard eye blinking, eyebrow-raising, jaw clenching, muscle tensing, eye-rolling, tensing individual muscles, joint clicking, finger bending, nose twitching, neck twisting, throwing the neck back, facial grimacing, lip smacking, and putting the chin down.

Complex Vocal Tics: Screaming, yelling words and phrases, saying sentences, swearing, mimicking noises, doing different accents, speaking in a made-up language.

Complex Motor Tics: Putting buckets on the head, snatching things and then giving them back, throwing things, doing yoga poses, kissing walls, dropping to the floor, running, jumping, clapping, ritualistic movements, hitting out at people, kicking, dancing, hitting oneself, jumping off of things, doing the middle finger, hopping.

Coprolalia: Coprolalia is the term for vocal tics that are socially inappropriate or obscene, this can include involuntary swearing. They can be as short as one word or they may be a few phrases at a time. They have no intention behind them just like all the other tics and they do not reflect our opinions or beliefs at all. Coprolalia tics can usually just be ignored as they are uncontrollable so it's important to accept it and understand that the person can't control it and is not choosing what they tic.

Management strategies like medication, therapy, or diet changes may be useful for some people but that is a personal choice and a medical professional or specialist can usually help a person find effective management strategies to deal with coprolalia and other tics. Coprolalia is the most stereotyped symptom of Tourette syndrome, it is said to affect only 10-15% of people with the condition, but it still needs more awareness as it's not as "funny" as the media portrays it as it can often be socially isolating. Some people may feel that their tics are trying to mortify them by saying the most inappropriate thing in any given situation. This can cause an individual to feel highly self-conscious.

Copropraxia: Copropraxia is the term for the involuntary use of inappropriate movements such as vulgar gestures and inappropriate touching, this is also a relatively rare tic but still needs more understanding as it isn't purposeful and is just from neurologically misfired signals.

Coprographia: This tic is where an individual may write or draw an obscene word or image uncontrollably. This can be very distressing for the individual, especially in school or work so it's important to be compassionate and understand that it isn't behavioral. Accommodations and support must be in place to make the workplace/school more accessible for the individual. Punishment, negative reinforcement, or even positive reinforcement will never reduce any tic, including these inappropriate tics. A person knows they are inappropriate but isn't able to stop.

Echolalia: Repeating the words and phrases of others.

Echopraxia: Repeating the movements of others.

Palilalia: Palilalia is where an individual may repeat certain syllables when trying to speak or keep starting a sentence over when trying to speak normally, this can sometimes look like a stuttering tic.

Phantom Tics: A phantom tic is where the premonitory urge before a tic is felt as an out-of-body sensation, this is said to be the rarest type of tic, although it may just be rarely spoken about as some people may conceal it due to the fear of being misunderstood or an inability to articulate how it feels. This sensation can occur before a complex motor tic or Tourettic OCD ritual and it can feel as if a clump of energy is engulfing objects and pulling the person towards it like an elastic band to perform a certain tic or ritual. Some people may feel very distressed when experiencing phantom tics as they are virtually unheard of and can be terrifying to experience. This fear can make it difficult to open up about it as people may not understand it and we may be afraid of being labeled 'crazy' when they are not, but this worry often leads to it being not very well known. A person may feel a phantom tic from the other side of the room, it isn't a thought, it is a physical sensation that seems to be projected onto the external environment. Some people may have phantom tics where they feel as if there's an invisible barrier in front of them and they may have to jump over it, some people may feel as if there is some sort of goo on their clothes and they may have to click it together until it "feels right." Some people may feel that there is a sensation on their hands that they have to wash off repeatedly. Other phantom tics may include feeling unable to touch certain objects as they may be contaminated by the sensation on top of them and some people may have tics where they feel as if they are being pinned down to the floor by this sensation and can't get up. Some people may feel it floating around them. For clarification, a phantom tic is different to an intrusive thought as it is a physical sensation and not an anxiety-driven thought, therefore CBT is usually ineffective for these tics and Tourettic OCD rituals and may make it worse due to the suppression elements. For some individuals who are severely impacted by these symptoms, these therapies may lead to rebounds and discomfort. If a child is asked about these tics then it may be described in a way that is difficult to understand, but this is because the individual is confused and overwhelmed and may refer to it as a made-up name such as "sticky magic".

Sensory Tics: A sensory tic is an involuntary sensation that can move throughout the body; however, it is different to a premonitory urge as it is not accompanied by a movement or vocalization. It isn't a warning that comes before a tic like a usual premonitory urge. It can feel as if there is a tic that is unable to escape the body, therefore it can be very distressing and uncomfortable. For some people, it may be likened to "itchy blood" and others may describe it as a feeling of pressure. Sensory tics may be triggered by tic suppression and an overload of tic triggers. These symptoms usually cannot be suppressed or redirected as they are automatic, they may cause an individual to become anxious and distressed due to the feelings it may cause. These sensations are physically intolerable and may be confused with extreme restlessness or even tactile hallucinations.

Self-injurious Tics: A self-injurious tic includes any tic that can harm the individual. This may include the individual hitting their own chest, scratching themselves or banging their head on something repeatedly.

Bladder Tics: A bladder tic is where a person involuntarily urinates as a tic. This can accompany a stomach-clenching tic. It can include small amounts of urine or the whole bladder emptying with force. The tensing of the abdomen can occur very suddenly and can be painful. Management of this tic can include wearing incontinence towels and adult diapers as well as managing pain where necessary through warm water bottles or warm baths if they are safe for the individual.

Bowel Tics: A bowel tic includes the involuntary excretion of feces, usually through tensing of the abdomen muscles and this can be very distressing and embarrassing to experience.

Breathing Tics: Breathing tics can include breathing in specific patterns, breath holding, forced exhalation and the feeling of not being able to satisfy the need to breathe. This can sometimes cause an individual to feel dizzy, lightheaded, and experience numbness in the extremities. A person will likely need to rest a lot when experiencing breathing tics.

Retching Tics: Retching tics are where an individual may vomit or gag uncontrollably, sometimes the urge for this tic may occur in the throat and can sometimes be managed by having a receptacle to throw up into. It can sometimes be dangerous as it can lead to malnutrition and not being able to digest medication because a person may keep hurling it back up due to the tic.

Writing Tics: This is where an individual may write (with pen, pencil or finger), type or draw something involuntarily.

Impulsive Tics: These are tics that could potentially have extremely dangerous consequences. These tics could include running into the middle of the road or trying to jump from a height. Again, these are involuntary tics and are not usually any indication of suicidal ideation unless other signs are present, but it is vital to talk to a professional about how to manage this perilous symptom. It can also help to talk to others in the Tourette syndrome community to see if any helpful coping mechanisms can be found to prevent harm from these tics.

Tic Attacks / Tic Fits: Sudden outbursts of extreme motor tics that can resemble seizures, dystonic episodes or full-body tremors. These tics occur pretty much non-stop and people may fall to the ground in these episodes. These may be accompanied by intense premonitory urges and severe non-stop vocal tics. They are different to non-epileptic seizures but they both look similar.

Mental Tics: Some people with Tourette Syndrome experience mental tics. These are where a person gets a random phrase, image, or string of numbers in the mind. Some people may have mental tics where they have to think of a certain word in their mind before they can say a word verbally, and some people may have random images pop up in their minds. Mental tics are slightly different to intrusive thoughts, as intrusive thoughts are fear and anxiety-based so the content of intrusive thoughts is usually dark and scary, but mental tics can be completely random and even happy thoughts. One example of a mental tic could be the word "cabbage" randomly popping into your mind every now and then, and another could be seeing a flash of artwork in your mind's eye every now and then. Intrusive thoughts, on the other hand, would be thoughts that scare you, and cause immense distress and anxiety because of the content in them. This isn't to say that mental tics can't be distressing, but they tend to be distressing for a different reason. Intrusive thoughts are distressing due to the content, but mental tics can just be distressing as the repetitive nature of the thoughts can be annoying and disruptive.

Observational Tics: Tics that comment on their surroundings and environment.

Visual Tics: These are tics that involve looking around in a certain way, such as needing to trace objects with the eyes due to a physical premonitory urge.

Dystonic Tics: These are tics that involve prolonged contraction or twisting of a muscle group. It can cause the muscles in that area of the body to feel tight and can restrict free movement. This is different from typical dystonia as dystonic tics can often be temporarily suppressed, but will happen again when a person isn't thinking about suppressing.

Tonic Tics: These tics involve the tensing of muscles and do not last as long as dystonic tics. Examples include a person tensing their buttocks for half a second, or tensing a muscle in their arm for around a second.

Clonic Tics: Clonic tics involve sudden jerking movements of a limb or body part. An example is if you suddenly had a tic that made you fling your arm out.

Belching Tics: These are tics that cause a person to burp. It may seem rude but the person doesn't mean to do it.

Remember that these are just examples. Not everyone will have all of these tics and there are also many other tics that cannot be included in this list - as anything can be a tic. Tics often change over time, so even if you haven't had a specific tic on this list, it doesn't mean that it isn't a possibility in the future. There is no one-size-fits-all all to Tourette Syndrome so everyone's experiences will be slightly different.

Many of the symptoms associated with Tourette's and other neurodivergent conditions can look very similar and can be confused with one another. For some people, it may not be necessary to distinguish between different symptoms, but some people feel that it is needed to determine which treatment option/management strategy may be the most effective if a particular symptom is causing distress or just for clarification, or to rule out any co-occurring conditions or a differential diagnosis.

How Do You Know If Something Is A Tic, a Stim, or a Compulsion?

Tics are the symptom that is most frequently associated with Tourette syndrome as tics are needed for a diagnosis, but other symptoms are usually present as well. Compulsions are usually associated with OCD or sometimes Tourettic OCD if it is a tic-like compulsion, and stimming is more associated with Autism but can also occur in Tourette Syndrome due to hyperactivity, anxiety, or sensory issues.

Stimming (also known as self-stimulatory behaviour) can include movements such as jumping, hand flapping, rocking backwards and forwards, swaying side to side, spinning, eye tapping, leg jiggling and more, vocal stims such as humming can also occur.

Tics:

- Tics are uncontrollable movements and vocalizations that can range from very mild to severely disabling.

- Almost any movement or vocalization that the body can physically do can be a tic.

- Tics often change over time and can be replaced by another within hours, days, weeks or years of it first appearing. Sometimes, when a person develops a new tic, it can be quite anxiety-provoking as they have no idea how long it is going to last, but the likelihood is that it will eventually pass and be replaced by other tics as time goes by.

- Tics can be simple or complex. Vocal tics can range from a subtle throat-clearing tic to a full sentence with linguistic meaning that may be in context, but it's vital to know that there is no intention behind it as people don't mean what they tic and it does not reflect the person's opinions as they don't choose their tics. Motor tics can range from a nose twitch to full body movements and repetitive ritualistic movements that must be performed in a specific order or until it 'feels right'.

- For many people, organic tics come with a strong, uncomfortable and distressing sensation beforehand, this is termed a 'premonitory urge'. This sensation can feel different for everyone. Some people describe it as an itch, a feeling of tension, pressure or 'itchy blood'. For some people, it may feel like there is something stuck to their skin or something stuck inside their throat or chest, and some people may feel the urge as a surge of electricity shooting up their spine or into their extremities. Different tics usually have different sensations, and the urge may be felt in a different part of the body from where the tic physically occurs.

- Tics often 'wax and wane' over time meaning that they can fluctuate in frequency and intensity, the periods of worsened tics may have a trigger such as certain dietary allergens, food additive sensitivities, fluorescent lights (photosensitivity), sensory overload, stress, excitement and anxiety. Some people can suppress their tics for certain periods of time; however, this should never be encouraged as it's very physically uncomfortable as the urge to tic builds up and can cause immense distress. The tics that are suppressed will always have to come out.

Stimming:

- Stimming is also known as "self-stimulatory behavior." The most common stims include rocking back and forth, swaying side to side, jumping up and down, hand flapping and hand wringing. Some people may have vocal stims as well.

- Stimming is usually repetitive and comes in bouts and is not necessarily as complex as tics. You won't just move your hands once as a stim, you'd flap them. You wouldn't just lean forwards as a stim, you'd rock back and forth. The less repetitive movements that do not come in bouts are more likely to be tics.

- Stims don't usually change much over time, a person will usually have similar stims throughout their life.

- Stimming usually happens when an individual is excited, when we are daydreaming about something that brings us joy, or listening to a piece of music that we love, we may feel a sudden burst of energy that comes out as stimming such as hand flapping or jumping up and down.

- Stimming can also help an individual to keep calm, a person may start stimming more when anxious or being overstimulated by sensory input, stims such as rocking back and forth can sometimes help people to stay calm. Tics are not an emotional regulation tool like stimming can be, despite the fact that tics do often get worse with stress, anxiety, and excitement as well.

- Stimming doesn't usually have an accumulating premonitory urge before it, it is possible to stop stimming but we should never be asked or encouraged to stop healthy stims as they help us to express and manage our emotions and regulate sensory input. Being told to stop stimming may trigger meltdowns as we are unable to let out our extra energy.

- Stimming can release beta-endorphins that can be beneficial to a person's well-being. Tics are more likely to cause distress. People often find stimming fun (but not always), but tics are not likely to be a source of fun or joy like stimming can be. This doesn't mean that the content of certain vocal tics can't be entertaining though.

- Stimming is usually associated with Autism (ASD) but can also occur frequently in people with sensory processing issues, anxiety, Tourette's, ADHD and more.

- Everyone in the general population stims in some way, such as hair twirling or leg shaking, but not everyone tics.

Compulsions:

- Compulsions are one of the main symptoms of Obsessive Compulsive Disorder. Something is typically a compulsion if it is fueled by anxiety or fear, or done in response to an intrusive thought in order to "neutralize it" or prevent something bad from happening.

- A person usually knows that their compulsions are irrational, but struggles to stop themselves from doing them due to intense anxiety.

- In classic OCD, suppression of compulsions can cause intense anxiety, but will eventually pass to the point where a person doesn't feel like they need to perform the compulsions as much. This must be done gradually, and ideally with the help of an ERP therapist. Suppression of tics won't cause fear, but will cause physical discomfort.

- Specific compulsions tend to happen in specific situations. For example, a person may have a compulsion that only happens when they are about to get into a car where they have to touch the windows in a certain way. Or, they may have a compulsion that only happens when they are getting ready for bed, where they have to flick the light switches on and off a specific number of times. Some tics may only happen in specific environments as well, but specific rituals may only occur in specific environments such as when using the bathroom, or trying to turn on a light switch.

In conclusion: Tics are not used as an emotional regulation tool and do not help a person manage sensory overload like stimming can be. Tics are not an emotional expression like stimming can be, though often do get worse with certain emotional states. Tics are not fuelled by anxiety or intrusive thoughts like classic OCD rituals are.

Everything You Need To Know About Vocal Tics

1) Vocal tics can be long and complex phrases, they can be in context and they can have a linguistic meaning so sometimes may look purposeful, however, they are still completely involuntary. The human brain is an incredibly complex organ, therefore tics can be very complex. If you hear someone yelling a whole phrase that may be in context, please know that this is still a tic and you should trust us as we know what is a tic and what is not. Some of us are wrongly accused of faking our condition as our tics can be extreme, but we shouldn't be judged like that. It's important to understand the complexity of the condition and that these tics are not purposeful.

When I say that tics can be in context, I mean that they may occur at good timing or may be situational.

2) We do not choose what we tic, if we could tic non-offensive things instead of having Coprolalia, then we would, but unfortunately, we don't really have a say in what comes out. I describe it like my brain has a 3-year-old inside that just wants to mortify me by making me tic whatever I shouldn't yell in a specific situation.

3) Vocal tics don't have volume control, people have asked me if I can whisper my tics or do them quietly, but that's not an option. If we could whisper our tics instead of screaming them at the top of our lungs in public, then we

would, but that doesn't happen as tics are involuntary and we don't choose the volume. If someone asks us to tic quieter, then we may end up ticcing louder. This is in no way, shape or form related to us being obnoxious. Instead, it is related to the fact that we are then focusing on the tics more and feeling more self-conscious, which can make them worse. The tics may also do the opposite of what we 'should' do in a situation so if we feel that we are meant to be quiet then the tics may be loud.

4) I know that in the media, the portrayal of Tourette's mainly focuses on Coprolalia (inappropriate tics) but it gives an inaccurate depiction of it. On television it's often portrayed as 'funny', but in reality, it isn't as funny as presented as coprolalia and other tics are often isolating and have many negative social implications. We often face harsh judgment, ridicule and discrimination from those who don't understand these symptoms. Coprolalia needs accurate depictions, despite it only affecting a small percentage of people with Tourette's, it still has a profound impact on the lives of those who experience it.

5) Please don't get offended by our tics as we cannot control them and they have no intention behind them, they are involuntary and not directed at anyone or anything. Sometimes, being met with offense can make us feel guilty for something we can't help. Understanding is vital and I'd like people to know that we don't mean what we tic. They don't reflect our views so please try not to get offended as it isn't us saying these things. When people are offended by us we can become very upset and withdrawn.

6) We are not thinking what we tic. Some of us may sometimes get an uncontrollable thought that comes into our mind before the tic comes out, like an intrusive thought, but it doesn't reflect our opinions at all. I'll often be thinking to myself "Don't tic that, don't tic that, don't tic that" and it goes around in my head on loop and then I'll unintentionally blurt it out as a tic. As it doesn't reflect our viewpoints or opinions, it's not what we are really thinking. It's more that we may involuntarily tic what we shouldn't or don't want to say in any given situation.

7) There is such a thing as observational tics where our tics uncontrollably comment on the environment around us. For example, if we see someone with a unique hair color then we may accidentally point it out and we may involuntarily comment on someone's weight or appearance, but we do not mean it. It has no intention behind it and it doesn't reflect what we really think. Our tics are just trying to mortify us. It can seem quite impulsive as it blurts out unwanted phrases in the worst situations. They are not directed at anyone, they are just set off by certain stimuli in our surroundings - such as things we see, hear, smell, or feel.

8) Some tics can occur once and then never happen again and can take us by surprise, tics are usually said to be repetitive movements and sounds which is true to an extent, but some tics can happen out of the blue and may not have any repetitive nature. This can be the case for some observational tics or random phrases which can be a one-off.

9. Sometimes, Coprolalia can occur mid-sentence and in context. For example, someone may be talking about their cat and may say "My fu**ing cat" when they meant to say "my cat". This can sound like they are saying it naturally as part of the sentence, but it is a tic. People may also add a swear word or insult onto the end of a sentence, for example, they may intend to ask someone "How was your day?" but it can come out as "How was your day Bi*ch?"

10) Tics are not a behavioral problem and should NEVER be punished. You cannot discipline the tics out of someone and those of us with Coprolalia (socially inappropriate and obscene tics) likely know that what we are ticcing is not appropriate, but we have no control over it.

11) Tics can sometimes occur in a different tone of voice to how we usually speak. It is common for some people to have a slightly more high-pitched or shrill voice when they tic, but people can and do tic in their normal voice as well.

12) Sometimes we may laugh about our own vocal tics as we can be surprised by the random and creative phrases they blurt out.

13) Sometimes our vocal tics are more about how a word feels than how it sounds. Our tics sometimes have to satisfy a premonitory urge, which is a physical sensation that some people feel before a tic occurs, and to do this the tic may have to feel a certain way when it is done. Some people may have lots of tics that come out with a

lot of force, as they need to satisfy the urge to tic. Some people may have tics which focus a lot on one specific sound or syllable. For example, someone may have lots of tics that have a "K" sound in as that is what the brain may involuntarily make someone say to satisfy the premonitory urge.

14) Please do not judge us as a person or make assumptions about our character based on what we tic. The kindest, sweetest, most caring person could have the most harsh tics towards someone they love (tics can be aimed at certain people but this is not done intentionally and is not within the person's control.) Someone with a brilliant work ethic may have very defiant and rebellious tics. Our tics are not a reflection of our character. Get to know us as a person rather than just getting to know the tics.

15) Tics can say other people's names so it can look like someone is directing a tic towards another person even though they don't want to direct their tics towards anyone.

This is a neurological condition, not a lack of willpower. Stop blaming yourself.

Chapter Three

MANAGEMENT STRATEGIES

Management Strategies For Tics

There are many options when it comes to managing tics, such as medications, supplements, therapies, lifestyle changes, dietary changes, and more used in the hope of reducing tics. In this chapter, we will be exploring those options.

Traditional Management Strategies:

Therapy: There is a therapy called Comprehensive Behavioral Intervention For Tics (CBIT) that is designed specifically to reduce the intensity of tics in those with conditions such as Tourette Syndrome. CBIT consists of three main elements - tic redirection, psychoeducation, and exposure with response prevention.

Tic redirection involves either fulfilling the urge to tic in another way that isn't as intense as the original tic - replacing the tic with a more subtle movement or vocalization that can still relieve the urge, or using a tic blocker which is a movement that stops the tic from being able to occur. Tic redirection can be helpful for people who have repetitive painful or dangerous tics as they may be able to replace the painful or harmful tic with something that doesn't hurt or cause problems.

Psychoeducation will help a person understand their condition and their triggers. However, some professionals may not fully grasp how it feels to have tics, so being taught about tics from someone who has never experienced them may backfire if the professional gets something wrong due to not experiencing tics themselves, this is why some people prefer to get the psychoeducation aspect through support groups where they can learn from other people who experience tics and talk to them about how they manage and how it feels for them.

The exposure-response prevention aspect is controversial as it can have the same effect as tic suppression. Many people find that tic suppression is uncomfortable and sometimes even painful. Many people struggle to focus when suppressing tics as all of their focus is going towards bottling up misfired neurological signals. As well as this, many people find that when tics are suppressed, they come out worse later on. Many therapists will disagree with this, but many people with Tourette syndrome do report outbursts of tic attacks and other symptoms such as rage attacks triggered by tic suppression.

Many people find that once they stop suppressing tics, they no longer have these severe episodes and outbursts. Holding in tics and "getting used to the urge to tic" as is encouraged in ERP can cause someone to stop listening to their bodies and may send the message of "you should live with uncomfortable and painful sensations (premonitory urges) and just get used to it so that you aren't an inconvenience to others". This is a very harmful message to send to someone. The individual's comfort and wellbeing should be paramount and a person should never be pressured to suppress symptoms or "normalize" themselves just to make other people more comfortable. Some people find the ERP aspect helpful in delaying certain tics so that they can be redirected. For example, if a person has an impulsive tic where they reach out and touch the stove, they may be able to learn to delay the tic so then it can then be redirected to prevent injury.

CBIT can be very helpful and life-changing for some people, but there is no size fits all so it won't work for everyone. It is seen as the first-line intervention when it comes to managing tics, but people with more complex tics and co-occurring conditions will likely need other interventions as well such as medications and/or lifestyle changes.

Below are some reasons why CBIT may not be effective for some people:

- Some people may not be able to feel their premonitory urges that come before tics. In this case, it is very difficult to redirect as you do not know how to fulfill an urge that you can't actually feel. As well as this, people may not even be aware that a tic is coming so they may not know when to implement tic blockers.

- On the other hand, some people may experience the opposite, where their premonitory urges are so strong that trying to satisfy them with a more subtle movement or vocalization just isn't possible. For some people, the premonitory urge that comes before a tic is more uncomfortable than the tic itself. For some ticcers, CBIT may help them cope with the uncomfortable feelings so that they blend into the background and don't bother the individual as much anymore. However, for other people, it may cause them to focus on the premonitory urge too much to the point where it just feels like it is becoming more intense and therefore more distressing.

- If people have too much of the ERP element, it may have a similar effect to tic suppression and just leave a person unable to focus on anything else other than managing the tics, which may make it difficult for a person to focus on their school work, for example. It may also create a rebound effect that there are many anecdotal reports of, where the tics actually end up exploding later on in the day after suppressing.

- If the therapist performing the psychoeducation aspect isn't actually a specialist in Tourette's, then they may miss out on some important information or spread misinformation. It has been documented that people have been told "writing tics don't exist" when they actually do, for example. Some doctors will also say that violent tics don't exist, despite the fact that many people have tics where they accidentally hit out at people or throw whatever is in their hands uncontrollably. Due to this, it is vital to find a therapist who actually specializes in Tourette Syndrome and who understands how complex tics can actually be.

Despite the fact that CBIT isn't a good fit for everyone, it is important to remember that some people do find it helpful in reducing problematic tics and it can get some people back into school or work if their tics are that bad that they struggle to cope in that kind of environment. CBIT has mixed reviews with some saying it really helped them and gave them their life back, and others saying it made matters worse.

Medications:

If therapy doesn't work for a person, or if it isn't enough on its own, then a person may be offered medication to help manage their tics. There isn't a medication that has been specifically designed just to treat Tourette Syndrome, but many medications are often used with success. Many of these medications come under the class of "antipsychotics", but despite the fact that they are designed to treat psychosis, they can also reduce tics for some people.

List Of Medications That May Be Prescribed For Tic Management:

Clonidine: Clonidine, also known as Catapres, is commonly used to treat migraines and high blood pressure. In some cases, however, it is also prescribed to manage tics. Clonidine is a vasodilator, meaning that it can lower blood pressure. This medication is also known to help manage the symptoms of ADHD, which commonly co-occurs with Tourette Syndrome. Clonidine is often trialled before antipsychotics in the management of TS as Clonidine is thought to have less of a risk of serious side effects. Antipsychotics work for Tourette's by reducing dopamine, but Clonidine works in a different way - it inhibits the release of norepinephrine. This medication is usually preferred for the management of mild to moderate tics, rather than for severe tics.

Common side effects from clonidine include feeling dizzy when standing up, feeling tired and weak, having a dry mouth, having headaches, feeling depressed, and experiencing constipation.

Topiramate: Topiramate, also known as Topamax, is an anti-epileptic medication. As well as being used to manage Epilepsy, it can be used for migraines and Tourette Syndrome. This medication does not work on the dopamine pathways, but instead normalizes nerve activity and calms overexcited brain signals. Possible side effects from this medication include hair loss, anxiety, cognitive problems, language problems, blurred vision, increased eye pressure, clumsiness, dizziness, confusion, concentration problems, abnormal appetite, mensuration problems, and tingling sensations.

Antipsychotics / Neuroleptics:
Antipsychotics, also known as neuroleptics, are often used in the management of Tourette Syndrome. Despite the fact that tics are not a form of psychosis, antipsychotics can help by reducing dopamine which is thought to be elevated in certain parts of the brain in Tourettic individuals. Below are some examples of antipsychotics that may be prescribed for the management of Tourette Syndrome and other complex tic disorders.

Risperidone: This medication is licensed to treat Schizophrenia, mania, and psychosis but can also be used to manage tics in Tourette Syndrome, severe OCD, and irritability in Autistic people. Risperidone works by reducing the levels of dopamine in the brain. It is an atypical antipsychotic which means that it has fewer side effects than typical ones. Side effects can include tiredness, Parkinson's-like symptoms, movement problems, weight gain, nausea, headaches, and increased levels of a hormone called Prolactin which can cause breast growth (even in males) and milk leakage out of the breasts.

Aripiprazole: This medication can be used to manage Schizophrenia, Bipolar Disorder, Tourette Syndrome, Depression doesn't get better with antidepressants alone, irritability, and behavioral problems. Some possible side effects from this medication can include headaches, dizziness, constipation, restlessness, weight gain, arm and leg pain, increased salivation, fatigue, uncontrollable twitching and jerking movements, anxiety, blurred vision, lightheadedness, nausea, abdominal pain, and sleeping problems. Aripiprazole is unique as it has the ability to both block and stimulate dopamine depending on how much is in the brain - it simply stabilizes dopamine levels. It is less likely than other antipsychotics to cause weight gain. It is a third-generation antipsychotic, meaning that it is newer and designed to cause fewer side effects.

Olanzapine: This medication is thought to be helpful for reducing tics and rages in people with Tourette Syndrome. Like other antipsychotics, it is traditionally used in the management of Schizophrenia and Bipolar Disorder. Olanzapine works by blocking dopamine receptors and altering serotonin levels in the brain. Weight gain is a common side effect of this medication. Other side effects are known to include swelling of the arms, face, hands, and feet, vision changes, speaking and swallowing problems, loss of balance, restlessness, tic-like movements in the face, and movement problems.

Haloperidol: This is a first-generation antipsychotic which has been used for Tourette Syndrome since the 1960s. Newer antipsychotics are generally preferred over Haloperidol as they are thought to have fewer side effects, but this medication is still sometimes used in the management of severe Tourette's. It is also thought that this medication may reduce feelings of anxiety. Possible side effects include problems speaking, issues with swallowing, muscle spasms, difficulty moving the eyes, severe and distressing restlessness, and weakness of the arms and legs. This medication is also known to cause weight gain.

Pimozide: This is a medication used for severe cases of Tourette Syndrome in order to reduce tics. It is not intended to be used as a first-line intervention and is reserved for those whose tics are severely disabling. Side effects from this medication may include difficulty speaking, dizziness, a high heart rate, a shuffling walk, loss of facial expression, stiffness in the extremities, breast swelling, the secretion of breast milk, and hand tremors.

Side effect lists are not exhaustive, others can occur, so speak with your doctor if you notice any strange symptoms appearing after starting a medication.

This is not an exhaustive list, but are just some examples of medications that are commonly prescribed to individuals with Tourette Syndrome. Any side effects should be reported to the prescribing doctor, but rest assured, there are many people who do not experience any side effects. Many people with TS find that medication changes their life for the better.

There is a very small risk of dangerous long-term effects or fatal side effects from antipsychotics, though these are exceedingly rare. Dangerous side effects can include:

Neuroleptic Malignant Syndrome: This is a life-threatening reaction to antipsychotic medication that can cause a fever, elevated heart rate, blood pressure fluctuations, mental status changes, muscle stiffness, excess saliva secretion, delirium, rapid breathing, and muscle tremors. Do be aware, however, that this condition is extremely rare and very unlikely to happen with the low doses of neuroleptics given to manage TS.

Tardive Dyskinesia: This is a condition caused by the use of antipsychotic medication. It is a movement disorder characterized by completely involuntary movements and twitches, such as tongue movements, lip smacking, excessive blinking, puffing out the cheeks, jaw movements, hip movements, arm movements, neck twisting, and jerking movements in the hands and legs. These may be mistaken for tics. Tardive Dyskinesia usually develops after taking antipsychotics for a long time. In some cases, Tardive Dyskinesia doesn't go away even after stopping the medication. Do be aware though, that this is a relatively rare side effect so many people do not go on to develop it.

Surgical Intervention For Tourette's:

Deep Brain Stimulation: DBS is a form of brain surgery where electrodes are implanted into the brain in an attempt to block the tic signals. It is not available in the United Kingdom at the time of writing this book, but is available in countries such as America. It is only used in extremely severe cases of Tourette Syndrome that do not respond to other interventions. This surgery can reduce the impact of tics for some people, and can also reduce OCD symptoms. It can however, cause complications such as serious infections, strokes, and reductions in speech fluency.

Natural and Alternative Management Strategies:

Many people choose to use natural and alternative management strategies if they do not respond well to therapy or medications, have unbearable side effects from medications, or just prefer to go down the natural route rather than the traditional path.

Diet Changes: Many people in the Tourette Syndrome community report that certain foods can make their tics worse. (Ludlow and Rogers, 2017) Some of the most common being caffeine (Müller-Vahl et al., 2008), food dyes, sugar, MSG, and artificial sweeteners. It appears that artificial food additives don't mix well with a highly sensitive nervous system.

There are many people who share their experiences online about how foods impact their tics. Online blogs and forums are filled with stories from people who have found natural ways to manage their tics, including through dietary changes. Even people with very severe tics have reported success through dietary interventions.

A study performed in 2018 showed that a gluten-free diet can be helpful for some people with TS. (Rodrigo et al., 2018)

Many people with Tourette Syndrome have high levels of inflammatory cytokines and other immune abnormalities. Certain food sensitivities, usually IgG sensitivities which cause delayed reactions, have been reported to exacerbate tics in some people. It could be that the consumption of the foods which an individual is sensitive to could increase inflammation in the body, therefore worsening tics. Food sensitivities which have been said to increase tics for some people include dairy, gluten (non-coeliac gluten sensitivity), corn, chicken, citrus fruits, nightshade vegetables, chocolate and salicylates. The foods which trigger tics in one person will not be the same as the foods that trigger tics in another. Everyone is different.

Some people will find out which foods trigger tics with the help of an environmental physician, naturopath, nutritional therapist, or functional medicine doctor. Some people just find out what foods make their tics worse through experience, where they notice a pattern over time. Some people discover that diet has an impact on their tics through an elimination diet, and some people will find out through IgG food sensitivity testing (but it is important to know that questions have been raised about the accuracy of these tests, they're not scientifically validated - though some people report that they have been helpful.)

Diets for Tourette Syndrome are incredibly understudied, yet people who do not respond well to therapy or medication may feel like they have no other option. Therefore, they may try diet changes as they have nothing to lose. One book which I would recommend that delves deep into the role of foods triggering tics is "Stop Your Tics By Learning What Triggers Them" By Sheila Rogers Demare.

Gerrard, Richardson, and Donat (1994) looked at 3 patients with movement disorders that were fuelled by the consumption of certain foods. Their movements all resembled tics, and each subject reacted to different food substances. This shows how different people react to different things.

ADHD is a common comorbidity of Tourette Syndrome, and interestingly, studies have shown that hypoallergenic diets can be helpful in reducing problematic ADHD traits. Dölp et al (2020) found that reduced ADHD rating scale scores could be seen in study participants on a hypoallergenic diet. Hypoallergenic diets can be difficult for some people with ADHD to follow though as they may struggle to prepare food due to executive dysfunction and may struggle with co-occurring eating disorders.

It is also possible that some people may have unique

genetic SNPs which cause their body to process certain nutrients differently. Nutrient processing issues can prevent the body from being able to create adequate levels of certain neurotransmitters, as it doesn't have the building blocks to do so. Many functional medicine doctors and nutritional therapists (not dieticians) utilize SNP testing in their practices.

On my YouTube channel, titled "Chronic Advocate", I created a video called "Diet for Tics? [In Tourette's & Related Conditions]" where I talk about the evidence that the food we eat may play a role in tic severity and frequency. I suggest that people watch that video if they would like to hear more on this topic and see examples of how people can be impacted by this.

If you as a parent decide that you would like to cut certain foods out of your child's diet to see if it reduces tics, it is vital to explain to the child that foods aren't "bad", but that you are just trying to help them have a better quality of life by making sure they aren't sensitive to certain foods. Explaining that food itself isn't "bad" can prevent a child from developing an unhealthy relationship with food.

It is also important for parents to explain to their child that they are not using any intervention to "normalize" them, as your child isn't broken and they need to know that they are loved and accepted as they are. Parents need to instead explain that these interventions are used to increase the child's quality of life, improve their well-being, and help them feel better. The intention should never be to try to get someone to fit into a neurotypical box for the sake of it, the intention should be to help the individual feel better and have a better quality of life. Before starting any major dietary changes, it is advisable to seek the insight of an environmental physician, naturopath, nutritional therapist, or integrative medicine doctor who has experience working with neurodivergent people. As well as advising you on how to find triggers and go about any necessary eliminations, they may also be able to help by recommending supplements to prevent deficiencies that could potentially arise from eliminating certain foods from the diet. Conventional dietitians aren't usually helpful when it comes to diets for neurological conditions, so you'll usually have to look outside of the conventional medical system for help with this.

Do be aware that dietary interventions won't work for everyone, the same as how there isn't one specific medication that works for everyone with TS, but no one would ever know if it could help them unless they try. If you're upset that you aren't responding well to medication or therapy, then it is important for you to know that there is still hope as alternative interventions may help.

Supplements: Magnesium is a nutritional supplement that is often mentioned in the Tourette Syndrome community. Some people find that it reduces the severity of their tics and eases feelings of anxiety. In fact, a few studies have been published on the role of Magnesium in Tourette Syndrome, many of which can be found in online databases. Magnesium mixed with vitamin B6 has been found to be helpful for some people with TS. (García-López et al., 2008).

Some people report that supplements which have anti-inflammatory properties can be helpful. This may be because people with Tourette Syndrome and co-occurring OCD can have higher levels of pro-inflammatory cytokines (Gabbay et al., 2009) and it is possible that reducing this inflammation may reduce the tics and related symptoms. Overactive immune responses involving both the innate and adaptive immune systems have been seen in some with TS. (Martino, Zis and Buttiglione, 2015)

Sensory regulation: Many people with Tourette's struggle with sensory processing issues. Some people with Tourette Syndrome have a co-occurring condition called Irlen® Syndrome (visual stress). There have been some reports of people who have both TS and Irlen® Syndrome who have seen a reduction in tics when wearing precision-tinted Irlen® lenses. As well as this, tics are known to get worse when a person is stressed or overstimulated. By giving someone the sensory tools that they need such as ear defenders or sunglasses, it may reduce feelings of overstimulation and therefore reduce tics. Having a dimly lit space that you can go to when having a severe tic episode may be helpful. Some people find it helpful to adjust clothing in a way that won't trigger tics. For example, if you find it uncomfortable to wear a tie to school to the point where it is exacerbating neck tics, you may be given permission to not wear a tie to school. This would be a reasonable adjustment and could help you focus more in lessons.

Taking part in activities of interest: Some people find that when they take part in an activity they're interested in and which takes a lot of focus, their tics temporarily reduce or even stop. Activities which people may find have this effect include singing, playing a musical instrument, doing a sporting activity, doing art, dancing, working on computer programming, or doing photography. Many people with Tourette's have at least one of these areas of interest that temporarily reduce their tics when focused on. This can be used to your advantage as it can help you cope with bad tic days and can allow you to become extremely talented in your areas of interest.

Epsom salt baths: These can help calm the muscles and reduce pain from tics.

Padded gloves: These can reduce the impact of self-injurious tics and punching tics by softening the area to prevent injury.

Extra tough furniture: People with very severe tics may need extra tough furniture to prevent the tics from breaking items around the house.

It is important to note that management strategies shouldn't be forced upon a person with Tourette Syndrome in an effort to "normalize" them, they should be used to improve a person's quality of life. Intention matters. If the person is old enough, they should ideally be involved in choices such as whether to start a new mediation or not.

Everyone's tic triggers are different. You will likely find your triggers over time. Keep an open mind.

Chapter Four

TIC SUPPRESSION

Tic Suppression

Some people have the ability to temporarily hold in their tics, known as tic suppression.

Some people may think 'if you can hold in your tics, then does that mean that you can control them?' The answer to this question is no - because although we may be able to temporarily stop our tics from showing, the underlying urge to tic and the misfired signals from the brain are still there. We are just masking it and bottling it all up. This causes the suppressed tics to accumulate, which is why many people report that tic suppression makes them worse.

Suppression can cause symptoms to present differently in different environments. Someone may tic frequently at home as they are letting their tics out freely, but may not appear to tic much at school as they are suppressing their tics.

Tic Suppression is Different From Tic Redirection and it is Different From Managing Tics and Reducing Them in Healthy Ways:

Tic suppression is where tics are forcefully held in without anything to help manage them, they build up and accumulate.

Tic redirection is where another action replaces a specific tic. A competing response is sometimes done to stop a harmful tic from occurring. The tic is either blocked or done in a different way, so that the urge is still satisfied but so that the tic doesn't cause harm. People may learn to redirect tics that cause injury or a lot of distress if they have the ability to do so.

Tic redirection is a healthy way to manage certain tics for many people, but there are also other ways to manage tics, such as medication and the elimination of triggering factors. These methods aren't the same as forceful suppression, as something is done to reduce the tics in the first place so that they may not need to be suppressed as much – the brain may not misfire as many signals when these interventions are used, so this isn't bottling the tics up, but genuinely reducing them.

The Rebound Effect:

Many people with tics report that they experience an explosion of more severe tics after suppressing them. This is known as the rebound effect. This explosion of more intense tics after suppression can be dangerous, as these severe tics may be destructive towards the person's surroundings and their own body which can lead to injuries. Many people report that they experience tic attacks triggered by tic suppression. Tic attacks are episodes of tics which are more intense than a person's usual level of ticcing, tic attacks from the outside may resemble seizures or dystonia, and a person's whole body may contort, jerk, and spasm.

Rage attacks are another symptom which people in the community sometimes report as being triggered by tic suppression. People have also reported that tic suppression has led to an increase in OCD symptoms and a decline in mental well-being in their case.

Many psychologists will state that they do not believe in the rebound effect, but this contradicts the experiences of countless people with Tourette Syndrome. Studies in this area are often overly generalized and may not take into consideration what a person with Tourette's experiences a few hours after suppression, as sometimes the rebound effect can be delayed and occur in the evening when a person is trying to relax. It has been noted that people with severe tics are sometimes turned away from these kinds of studies, so it isn't right for the results to be generalized to everyone with TS.

Furthermore, it is possible that the psychologists in charge of these studies may have found a way to manipulate results in order to get the findings that they want. There is a particular conflict of interest if they perform behavioral interventions for tics such as ERP as a career, as they will want the findings to promote their work and make it seem like there are no risks or ethical issues to what they are doing. Please also remember that these therapists have usually never experienced tics themselves, therefore they can't imagine what it really feels like to have to suppress tics.

Statistics:

In a poll, I gathered the following statistics:

For the question "Do you think tic suppression is unhealthy?"

- 93% said yes.
- 7% said no.

For the question "Do you find that tic suppression makes your tics worse?"

- 96% of respondents answered 'yes'
- 4% answered 'no'.

124 people responded.

For the question "Do you think it is bad for people to be encouraged to suppress tics?"

- 93% of people answered 'yes'
- 7% answered 'no'.

131 people responded to this question.

The last two questions were only answered by people who had tics themselves.

What Does Tic Suppression Feel Like?

When people suppress their tics, the premonitory urge (the sensation that comes before a tic) may get stronger and stronger. It accumulates until it becomes physically intolerable. This is why some people say that tic suppression is painful for them and hurts. It may feel like a buildup of pressure inside of someone or an uncomfortable sensation on someone's skin or inside a certain part of their body.

Many people report that when they are suppressing tics, they may not be able to focus on much else except not ticcing. It can take up the majority of someone's mental focus, so the person may be unable to perform as well as usual in school or in the workplace if they are holding in their tics. Many people also report that tic suppression makes them extremely tired and tense.

Some people find that suppressing vocal tics makes them feel as if they can't breathe. The discomfort from suppressing tics can sometimes be worse than the tics themselves.

Subconscious Suppression:

Many people suppress their tics without even realizing they are doing it. This can happen in environments where a person has an underlying fear of being judged, bullied, or being seen as 'different'. Some people subconsciously suppress tics for their own safety in these situations, but it still isn't without risk.

Unlearning Tic Suppression:

Some people feel that those with tics should 'learn to suppress', but many people already subconsciously suppress, to the detriment of their own well-being. This is why many people try to unlearn tic suppression. People try to tic freely again after so many years of suppressing. This is so that they can experience better well-being, less tension in their bodies, and fewer negative consequences from suppressing the tics.

Our instinct to try and suppress our tics may be ingrained from early on in our tic journey, so unlearning suppression and doing what we feel is best for us can take time.

How Encouraging Someone To Suppress Their Tics Can Harm Their Self-Esteem:

When we are taught to hide or mask something which our bodies make us do automatically, we get the sense that our differences are 'bad'. We may feel a sense of shame for something we cannot control, as we have been taught to feel that way. We may feel ashamed of having neurologically misfired signals. Some people can't suppress their tics much at all, and this is okay, but when these people are encouraged to suppress their tics, they may feel as if they are 'weak' or 'lack self-discipline' or are being a 'rebel' when they experience their tics. This is extremely saddening.

Feeling like we have to suppress our tics can hinder our development of self-acceptance, and seeing as some people have tics their entire life, it's better to learn self-acceptance sooner rather than later.

We know how to suppress our tics, but it can be harmful, therefore many of us are forced to spend our adult years learning how to tic freely again.

Is Tic Suppression Ever Necessary?

Sadly, there can be situations where people don't really have a choice about whether they suppress or not. For example, if there is any risk of being a victim of violent hate crimes, fights, or bodily harm. Of course, for life-or-death situations and times where there is a risk of serious injury to someone - temporary suppression may be necessary. However, in most situations where there is no risk, suppression should be discouraged.

Affirmations:

- If people expect me to hold in my tics when it harms me, they do not accept me as I am, so I need to accept myself and do what is best for me.
- I am allowed to tic freely and let go of shame.
- My tics were never a lack of willpower, they are a neurological difference.

Your tics are the pathway to freedom, to allow you to be yourself in a society that tries to control you and dictate how you act.

Chapter Five

CO-OCCURRING CONDITIONS

Around 86% of people with Tourette Syndrome have another condition alongside it.

It is rare for Tourette's to occur alone. In this section, we will be covering some of the conditions which can co-occur with TS.

Attention Deficit Hyperactivity Disorder:

ADHD is a neurodevelopmental condition where a person experiences hyperactivity and/or a dysregulation of attention. If you have ADHD, you may feel restless, agitated, and unable to stay still. Individuals with ADHD may have racing thoughts which distract them from daily tasks. People may appear very 'absent-minded' as they struggle to pay attention to what they are doing. If you have ADHD, you may accidentally make a lot of mistakes in your work, or you may uncontrollably rush through things.

People may only be able to skim-read text rather than reading it in depth, as their brain won't let them pay attention for long to something that isn't fascinating.

People may struggle with forgetfulness, and may commonly lose items that they need, or may leave things where they are not supposed to be left, such as leaving the keys on the outside of the door or leaving the milk out of the refrigerator.

People with ADHD are likely to struggle with executive functioning skills, which are the mental skills needed to organize, prioritize and plan. Executive functioning is needed for someone to be able to think with flexibility, inhibit actions which are inappropriate, make decisions, regulate emotions, learn from past mistakes, initiate (start) a task, and predict the consequences of their actions.

Some people with ADHD experience Rejection Sensitive Dysphoria. This is where a person may have strong and unpleasant emotional and mental reactions to the perception of criticism, rejection, disapproval, or exclusion. Some people with the RSD aspect of ADHD may go above and beyond to avoid rejection or criticism, even if they end up overworking themselves to the point of burnout.

Sensory Processing Disorder: Sensory Processing Disorder is a condition where people have difficulty processing sensory input. Those with SPD may be over-sensitive or under-responsive to certain sensory input such as tastes, noises, textures and lights. Some people with Sensory Processing Disorder have vestibular processing issues. The vestibular sense is related to balance, so people may try to compensate for this and feel more at ease by rocking back and forth (commonly associated with Autism.) Some people may also have proprioceptive processing issues. Proprioception is the sense of where we are in space, and where different parts of our body are. Some people may also have interoceptive processing issues. This is the sense of what is going on inside of our body, such as being able to tell if we are hungry or not. People with this sort of processing issue may be unaware that they haven't had anything to drink all day, as their brains may not process the perception of thirst.

People with Sensory Processing Disorder may avoid certain sensory input and/or crave and seek certain sensory experiences.

Irlen® Syndrome: This is a condition associated with light sensitivity. People with this disorder may have difficulties reading as the text may become distorted or the contrast between white paper and black text may be too overwhelming or distracting.

Individuals with Irlen® Syndrome may struggle to comprehend what they are reading, particularly when under bright lighting. People with this condition may have other symptoms when under bright or fluorescent lighting, such as feeling agitated, tired, hyperactive, and being unable to concentrate. Some people with Irlen® Syndrome have major problems with depth perception when in a brightly lit room.

Some people with Irlen® Syndrome get headaches or migraines when they are under bright lights, and they may experience major discomfort when using electronic screens due to the light they give off.

Some people with Irlen's struggle to drive due to glare.

Irlen® Syndrome is not a problem relating to the eyes, but is the brain's inability to process certain wavelengths of light.

Some people with tic disorders report a significant reduction in tics when light sensitivity is addressed. This is because light can overwhelm the brain of a sensitive individual, in turn exacerbating the tics.

Most doctors have never heard of Irlen® syndrome (also known as Scotopic Sensitivity Syndrome or Visual Stress.) This is why it is important to find a certified Irlen® practitioner who can provide a screening. Some optometrists can perform an intuitive colorimeter test which can detect visual stress as well.

Reading difficulties associated with Irlen® syndrome (such as poor comprehension, visual distortions of text, and overpowering white glare) can be managed by using a tinted overlay that goes over the paper when reading. The tint needed will be different for different people.

If overlays are not enough, for example, if a person has abnormal perceptions of their environment, has constant over-active brain activity when under bright lights, or has migraines when under bright lights, then tinted Irlen© spectral filters may help. The tint needed will be different for each person and an assessment is necessary to determine the precision tint that will help the individual.

Autism Spectrum Condition: Autism Spectrum Disorder (also referred to as Autism Spectrum Condition) is a condition that affects every aspect of a person's life, but is primarily thought to affect social interaction and social communication. Autistic people often have a collection of traits such as being very sensitive to particular sensory input, getting overwhelmed and overstimulated easily, struggling to cope with daily life, having intense passions and areas of expertise (special interests) that consume a person's mind and attention, having high levels of anxiety, and stimming (which can include rocking backwards and forwards, jumping up and down, twirling, clapping, hand flapping etc). Stims are different to tics, though they can sometimes look similar.

Some Autistic people struggle with verbal communication and may be non-speaking or semi-verbal, however, a lot of autistic people do well with verbal communication but struggle more with non-verbal communication. In these cases, people are likely to struggle with reading social cues, understanding facial expressions, figuring out other people's intentions, making eye contact, knowing when it is their turn to speak, seeing other people's viewpoints and understanding sarcasm.

Every Autistic person is impacted differently.

Dyscalculia: Dyscalculia is a specific learning difficulty related to numbers and math computation. People with Dyscalculia are likely to be years behind what is expected in their mathematical performance. People with Dyscalculia may count on their fingers, be slower to work out the answers to mathematical equations, struggle to perform addition, subtraction and multiplication, and have difficulty memorizing mathematical facts.

People with Dyscalculia often experience high levels of math anxiety and may experience an avoidance of math topics, however, Dyscalculia isn't the same as math anxiety. The anxiety in people with Dyscalculia comes from the inability to understand arithmetic, whereas people can have math anxiety regardless of how good they are at maths.

Generalized Anxiety Disorder: GAD is a condition where a person feels excessively worried and nervous about many different things. People may feel tense, on edge, and afraid most of the time. People with GAD can have other symptoms such as getting tired more easily than other people due to frequent adrenaline surges, having trouble focusing due to frantic thoughts, experiencing irritability, and having physical symptoms from anxiety such as a racing heartbeat, stomach aches, and feelings of breathlessness. It is vital not to automatically assume that physical symptoms are caused by anxiety though as these symptoms can also be caused by a variety of other conditions such as dysautonomia, SIBO, etc. To be diagnosed with Generalized Anxiety Disorder, a person must have experienced anxiety symptoms for at least 6 months.

Functional Neurological Disorder: FND isn't always listed as a condition that commonly co-occurs with tic disorders, however, there are quite a lot of people who have both Tourette Syndrome and Functional Neurological Disorder.

FND is a condition where people experience neurological symptoms that are not due to a structural change in the brain or nervous system, but are due to the brain being unable to send the correct signals. FND can cause many symptoms and different people will have different ones. Some of the symptoms include seizures, paralysis, sensation changes, memory problems, speech problems, dystonia, muscle twitching, walking problems, and much more. The symptoms of FND are completely involuntary and can be disabling. Some studies link FND to inflammation. Kozlowska et al. (2018) and Van der Feltz-Cornelis et al. (2021) explored this.

Depressive Disorders: There are various types of depressive disorders such as Major Depressive Disorder and Persistent Depressive Disorder (Dysthymia). Major Depressive Disorder is a condition where a person experiences extremely low mood and a loss of interest in activities. People with Major Depressive Disorder often lose the ability to feel pleasure or joy from activities that once interested them. Major Depressive Disorder can be diagnosed once a person has had these types of symptoms for more than two weeks.

People with Depression often have other symptoms such as difficulty sleeping, loss of appetite, lack of energy, lack of ability to care for oneself, irritability, pessimistic thoughts, excessive feelings of guilt and shame, weight loss or gain, doing everything slowly, and sometimes - self-harm and suicidal thoughts.

Dysthymia is a condition where people experience a low mood that isn't intense enough to meet the criteria for Major Depressive Disorder, for most days for at least 2 years.

Many studies link the development of depression to inflammation, such Berk et al. (2013).

Dysgraphia: This is a specific learning difficulty that causes problems with handwriting. A person with Dysgraphia may have illegible handwriting and may write very slowly. People with Dysgraphia will often have problems when it comes to writing in a straight line, spacing letters evenly, and forming the shapes of letters. It is not a lack of effort, but is related to problems with motor coordination and visual processing. Punishing a child with Dysgraphia for having poor handwriting will not help, and will just lower their self-esteem. If you have Dysgraphia, you may struggle to keep your writing aligned with the margin of the page. It is important that if a decline in handwriting is seen at the same time as the onset of the tics, that PANDAS/PANS is considered as these conditions can cause both tics and handwriting decline to occur concurrently.

Pyrrole Disorder: According to articles written by Pyrrole experts, Pyrrole disorder is commonly seen in people with Tourette Syndrome. This is a condition characterized by having too many pyrrole molecules in the body. This can cause symptoms such as anxiety, irritability, rages, severe depression, sensory sensitivities, and an inability to cope with the stressors of daily life. Pyrrole Disorder is usually misdiagnosed as a mental health condition such as Bipolar Disorder, Depression, or Anxiety, which prevents people from getting the appropriate treatment. A functional medicine doctor, nutritional therapist, or naturopath may be able to check for Pyrrole disorder. Pyrrole disorder can also cause physical symptoms, such as morning nausea, frequent infections, bloating, irritable bowel syndrome, joint pain, and prominent stretch marks on the skin.

Pyrrole disorder can be diagnosed using a urine test, called the Kryptopyrrole test. Pyrrole disorder can't currently be treated with medication, but nutritional supplements can help. Symptoms of Pyrrole Disorder occur because the excess Pyrrole molecules bind to certain nutrients in the body such as zinc and vitamin B6, and they then get excreted through the urine leading to nutritional deficiencies. Without adequate nutrition, the body cannot create certain neurotransmitters.

Other Traits That People With Tourette's Can Experience:

It is vital to know that Tourette's is so much more than tics. As you have just read, it can co-occur with many other conditions, but people with TS can still have traits of OCD, ADHD, and SPD even without meeting the full diagnostic criteria for those conditions. These sub-clinical traits can still have an impact on a person's quality of life.

Rage attacks are a symptom experienced by around 40% of people with Tourette's, characterized by involuntary outbursts of aggression. This will be discussed more later on in this book.

Tourette's is a complex neurodevelopmental condition, and some of the other traits such as sensory issues or rages may impact a person more than the tics themselves so it is important not to ignore these symptoms.

Below is a list of other characteristics commonly experienced by Tourettic people:

Disinhibition: Some people with Tourette Syndrome struggle to inhibit certain impulses, even those that are not tics. For example, if there's a sign that says "do not touch" - a person with TS may touch it without even thinking, people may also be unable to inhibit emotional reactions such as excessive laughter, or sudden inappropriate remarks. People who experience disinhibition will usually know that certain actions are "socially inappropriate" but cannot take the time to stop themselves and think before doing something. They only realize they've done something "inappropriate" afterwards and may be confused as to why they did that.

Irritability: Although irritability is usually associated with PANDAS/PANS more than TS, many people with TS also struggle with feelings of irritability due to co-occurring ADHD, anxiety, sensory overload, and discomfort from tic urges as well as frustration related to being misunderstood all the time. It has been found that those with more severe tics (particularly vocal tics) often struggle more with irritability. (Cox and Cavanna, 2015)

Social differences: It is said that people with Tourette Syndrome can experience higher levels of social immaturity (which is spoken about in the article "Understanding Behavioral Symptoms in Tourette Syndrome" by the Tourette Association of America) and can also have lower levels of social skills. (Bitsko et al., 2020) According to a study from 2011, people with

Tourette Syndrome may perceive facial expressions slightly differently and also may perceive humor in a unique way. (Eddy et al., 2011) This does overlap with Autism, which can sometimes co-occur with Tourette syndrome. It is said that 1 in 5 children with Tourette syndrome meet criteria for Autism Spectrum Disorder. (Darrow et al., 2017)

Traits of personality disorders: A 1997 study found that out of 39 adult patients with Tourette Syndrome, 64% of them had one or more person-
ality disorder. (Robertson et al, 1997.) Cluster C Personality Disorders are thought to be the most common cluster in Tourettic people. Histrionic personality is said to be the rarest among Tourettic people.

Sensory sensitivities: It is thought that at least 80% of people with Tourette's report higher perception to sensory stimuli. It has also been found that faint repetitive or constant external sensory stimuli can be more bothersome to Tourettic individuals than more intense sensory stimuli. (Belluscio et al., 2011) People with severe sensitivities to sensory stimuli will often be diagnosed with Sensory Processing Disorder, however, sometimes a co-occurring diagnosis isn't necessary as these sensory sensitivities can just be seen as part of the spectrum of Tourette Syndrome.

You don't need to be neurotypical to be worthy of love.

Chapter Six

OBSESSIVE COMPULSIVE DISORDER

Obsessive Compulsive Disorder

OCD is such a complex and debilitating condition that I felt it needed its own chapter.

Around 60% of people with Tourette's have co-occurring OCD. OCD is an anxiety disorder where people experience uncontrollable and unwanted thoughts, known as intrusive thoughts. These thoughts are often the last thing a person would want to think and they can make a person feel intense shame, guilt, anxiety, distress and discomfort. The intrusive thoughts are often based on what a person is most against, meaning they are ego-dystonic. So a person who is highly religious or spiritual may involuntarily have blasphemous thoughts about God, a person who loves and cares about their family may have visions of killing their family members, and a person who is afraid of thinking negative thoughts may have a constant negative inner voice. These thoughts aren't really from them, it is from the OCD, but because the thoughts seem to the person like it is them really thinking those things they may feel like they're just a horrible person. These intrusive thoughts are a form of obsession. Other obsessions that can occur in those with OCD include worries and fears that consume a person's mind and may be all that a person thinks about. For example, a person may be so consumed by the fear of getting ill that they cannot stop thinking about it and spend hours of the day performing compulsions that they feel may reduce the chances of them getting ill, despite the fact that the person usually knows it is irrational. Other kinds of obsession can include urges, such as the unstoppable urge to keep things even and intense urges to perform various compulsions.

The compulsions that someone with OCD experiences may be extremely time-consuming, possibly taking between 1-15 hours out of the day. Compulsions can be overt or covert. Overt compulsions are ones where a person performs a physical action that is often visible to others, whereas covert compulsions are hidden. Covert compulsions are usually in the form of mental compulsions - rituals that occur in the mind. These mental compulsions can include affirming over the intrusive thoughts in the mind, ruminating to try and find an answer to something which is uncertain, checking one's own intentions or memories, repeating a certain word or phrase in the mind to reduce anxiety or trying to push away an intrusive thought, and more.

There are countless different OCD subsets / themes, here are some examples:

Morality / Scrupulosity OCD:

Morality / Scrupulosity OCD revolves around the fear of being immoral or not following a religion correctly. People with this OCD theme may obsessively follow religion to the point where it can become unhealthy, for example, praying for hours a day when other things need to be done or being afraid to do anything in case you "accidentally sin."

People may have an obsession with following the "right path" so that they can "do everything right" but this can leave people stuck, too afraid to make new decisions or move forwards in life out of fear of unintentionally doing something "immoral". They may obsess over every little decision in case it could send them down the "wrong path" and lead to them "going to Hell" or doing something bad.

- People may have intrusive thoughts that go against their morals, values and beliefs. For example, involuntarily thinking disrespectful things about God, having thoughts about sinning, or visualizing sacred texts being destroyed.

- People may pray excessively, opt out of making decisions as they don't know if it's 'right', read scriptures constantly, obsessively practice gratitude, ruminate about whether they may have done anything wrong and whether they have 'learnt their lesson', apologize constantly, obsess over whether they are doing, feeling or thinking the 'right thing', have an avoidance of religious or spiritual things as they know it will trigger the uncertainty and anxiety, or they may go to religious establishments very frequently etc. These are just some examples of how this subset of OCD may present.

- If a person does something that could be perceived as 'bad' or 'wrong' they may panic and feel very intense guilt and shame, out of proportion to the situation.

- People may live in fear of doing the wrong thing and may review every action they perform.

- People may research things about spirituality or how

to 'be a better person' and may try to excessively incorporate these characteristics into their daily lives or may fear that they won't incorporate them. They may feel intense shame for the times they haven't done these things in the past.

Sexuality OCD:

- This is characterized by intrusive thoughts and uncertainty about one's sexuality that is excessive and causes distress in daily life.

- This is different from someone wondering if they are genuinely a different sexuality, this is the inability to find certainty that causes immense distress.

- Some people may worry that by accidentally looking at someone's breasts, for example, would that mean that they are secretly a lesbian?

- People may just worry about the uncertainty, they may know their sexuality, but their OCD causes them to doubt it, making them question whether they are bisexual and just don't know it, for example.

- People with this form of OCD may have intrusive thoughts about same-sex relationships which can cause anxiety, but it should not be assumed that people with this form of OCD are homophobic as they can be very accepting of others' sexuality, they are just afraid of uncertainty and want a concrete answer so that they can solidify their sense of identity.

- People may have worries about whether they are gay and whether that will mean that they have to leave their wife and kids, for example, or they may worry that the way they are sitting makes them 'look gay' even though sexuality doesn't actually have a look.

- People in the LGBT+ community can also have sexuality OCD, and may worry about "becoming straight" as it could change their identity and sense of self.

- This isn't about someone genuinely questioning their sexuality, it is a full-on obsession that causes distress, a person may know they are straight but may still obsess over the possibility of being gay, or vice versa.

Relationship OCD:

- This subset often revolves around a fear that you may cheat on your partner, fall in love with another or secretly be in love with another person. People may worry whether they're good enough or if their partner is right for them. Some people may have doubts and worries about whether they really love their partner which can cause immense distress.

- It is normal to worry about some of these things sometimes, but with Relationship OCD, these worries can take hours out of a person's day.

- People may obsessively take relationship tests, read articles on relationships, or journal about their relationship to try and get some clarity, they may constantly ruminate about the relationship and whether it will work out and may try to figure out whether they are subconsciously in love with someone else. Some people may have the urge to break the relationship off, they may monitor their thoughts about the relationship, they may make comparisons with other people's relationships, and people may seek reassurance from their partner.

Existential OCD:

- The involuntary obsession over very deep questions such as ponderings surrounding the universe, why we are alive, the meaning of love, why we have gratitude, or how things in the world add up to make sense.

- People may ruminate for hours trying to find certainty, otherwise, it can feel as if everything is pointless. If you are plagued with these questions and cannot find an answer (as no one really knows it) then you may not see the point in doing anything or living your life.

- People may read countless articles or watch documentaries trying to find answers to their minds' questions.

- This is different from normal existentialism due to the frequency of these thoughts and the impact they have on someone's life, it can be debilitating. We all think about these questions from time to time, but for someone with this form of OCD they feel as if they NEED an answer.

It is not just curiosity in this case, it is desperation and means that the person may feel like they can't fully live their life without the answers.

OCD with covert compulsions / Pure-O OCD:

- This is where a person has intrusive thoughts and obsessions without outwardly obvious compulsions. The compulsions if present in this subset tend to occur in the mind (covert compulsions.)

- Some people with OCD may fear that having negative thoughts could cause bad things to happen, due to karma for example. It is important to know that everyone has negative thoughts and they do not really mean anything.

- Some people may argue with the intrusive thoughts inside their head, as the intrusive thoughts may seem like someone is saying something in the mind, but this is completely separate from a delusion as we know that it is just a thought and that no one is really in our mind.

- People may have mental compulsions where they try to erase the thoughts, apologize in their mind, pray in their mind, visualize something, do a mental ritual, repeat a mantra in their mind, affirm over the intrusive thoughts, try to rethink the thought without the bad thing happening and more...

- Having so many mental compulsions can make it virtually impossible to focus on your outside surroundings, so people may seem a bit 'spacey' or 'absent-minded' as their attention is focused on what is going on in their minds.

Sensorimotor OCD: This is an obsessive awareness of bodily functions such as breathing, swallowing or blinking. People may overthink these things and wonder whether they are breathing correctly or whether they are blinking too much, they may panic and worry about whether or not they will ever be able to stop focusing on these things.

Emotional / Mental Contamination OCD:

- This is the excessive worry that you may transmit negative emotions, thoughts, or energy to others, or that you will be contaminated with another person's negative feelings.

- People may feel that their "aura" or "essence" is contaminated and unclean from intrusive thoughts or feelings.

- Some people may feel that the idea of a certain person is contaminated, if they feel feelings of betrayal or disgust around a person, they may wash after being with that person, not touch that person's possessions, and avoid the person as the general idea of them or the emotions that they evoke can be seen as a contaminant.

- People may fear that by being around others with 'negative' personality traits, they may acquire these traits.

- People may avoid family members or friends and not go near them due to the fear of contamination from their "energy".

- Some people may have psychological feelings of 'dirtiness' that they may try to wash away.

- In severe cases, Some people may think that their emotions will contaminate the world and cause bad things to happen, this can make someone wonder whether the world would be better off without them as they worry that their emotional state may be linked to word events, and may worry about being responsible for these things due to how they feel.

Germaphobia / Contamination OCD:

- People may be absolutely terrified of germs, contamination or getting ill / becoming sick due to germ exposure.

- People may spend hours handwashing or take multiple showers or baths every day.

- People may change their clothes multiple times a day when they feel they have been 'contaminated'.

- People may not touch door handles or other things

that could be 'contaminated'.

- People may feel that if they have germs on them they may acquire a serious disease and this may consume a person's every waking thought.

- People may be afraid to breathe in certain places as they may feel that the air is 'contaminated'.

"Just right" OCD:

- This is the need for everything to be "just right" such as needing things to be symmetrical, needing to have objects in a certain place, evening things out, ordering things up, or lining things up perfectly. This is similar to perfectionism OCD except it has more to do with the placement of objects and a sensation of things being "just right" rather than pure anxiety.

- People may spend hours trying to align things or even them up, this can include shoes, pencils and pens, papers or other items. It can feel like there is a sensation around it, similar to Tourettic OCD, or that it just needs to feel 'right'.

- It can feel like it won't let you win, because if the object is straight then it is 'too perfect' but if it is wonky then it is 'not straight enough' so it goes on and on in this cycle but won't let you leave it alone as you are compelled to do it. OCD will do whatever it can to torment you and keep you doing rituals.

- Things may need to be in a certain place, or touched in a certain way.

- Socks may need to be the same height so that they are even, for example, people may spend ages trying to make sure they are equal.

Harm OCD:

- This subset revolves around the excessive worry that you may accidentally harm someone or that you may have harmed someone in the past without realizing it.

- You may have intrusive thoughts about harming those you love, sometimes the thoughts are violent and aggressive and you may worry about accidentally acting on these.

- You may worry that you're a vicious and aggressive person when you are really not.

- People may be terrified that they might hurt someone on impulse, or that they may be responsible for causing someone harm.

- People may hide dangerous items from themselves or avoid them such as knives, chemicals etc.

- Some people may also have intrusive thoughts about harming animals or themselves, and this can be incredibly distressing.

- A person may try to figure out whether they have anything in common with criminals or violent offenders. People may research this to try and find out.

- The person may review every action and play out past events in their mind to see if there is any way they could have caused harm, sometimes the mind can play tricks and the individual may be almost convinced that they harmed someone.

- They may seek reassurance from others as to whether they have harmed someone and "confess" thoughts.

- Some people may worry that by having these intrusive thoughts, it may harm the individual who is in the thoughts just by thinking it.

Time OCD:

- The obsession with presence, or wondering whether you are doing things too fast or slow.

- A person with Time OCD may obsessively try to be mindful or may keep checking the time. They may ALWAYS feel like they need to know what time things happen.

Checking OCD:

- This is where people may feel compelled to check things such as light switches to ensure that the light is off, they may check to ensure that the stove is off or that the door is locked, they may check an email repeatedly before they send it, they may re-read labels over and over again, they may check that their friend is still friends with them on social media, etc. This checking tends to happen for an excessive amount of time.

- Some people may have checking compulsions that others cannot see such as intention checking in an attempt to check in their mind that they have pure intentions and this can cause a lot of rumination, some people may have sensation-checking rituals where they check whether they are feeling any sort of unwanted attraction, Some people have emotion checking to see if they are feeling the 'right way' in a specific situation or to see if they have enough empathy, some people may check past events through rumination to ensure that they haven't missed anything, and some people may repeatedly recall information in their conscious mind to check that they haven't forgotten.

- Everyone checks things sometimes, but with this form of OCD, it is incredibly excessive and can take up a lot of someone's time, and most people would be able to brush these concerns off such as 'Did I turn the light off?' and they would be able to stop after one check, but someone with this form of OCD cannot stop thinking about it or obsessing over it. It causes immense distress and anxiety over something that wouldn't really bother people without the condition. No matter how many times they have checked, they are still plagued with doubt.

Tourettic OCD vs Classic OCD:

Most people in the general population and in the Tourette's community have Classic OCD. Classic OCD is characterized by having rituals that are fueled by anxiety, intrusive thoughts and fear. For example, someone may open and close the door repeatedly as their mind tells them that their family will die if they don't. Although Classic OCD is what most people know of, there is a subset called Tourettic OCD that doesn't tend to follow the same pattern.

In Tourettic OCD, the rituals are fueled by physical sensations and a need to get a "just right" feeling, rather than by anxiety or fear. In Tourettic OCD, a person may open and close the door repeatedly as they have a phantom tic making it feel like there is a blob of energy stuck on the door, they may perform the ritual until the "blob of energy" feels like it falls off.

Another example of a Tourettic OCD ritual could be someone pushing their arms against a car window and having to click their fingers, then smear their arms down the glass pane. The individual may have to repeat this every time they get into a car. Due to the repetitive nature of this happening only in a specific situation, having to be completed in a specific way, and being ritualistic – it looks like an OCD ritual. However, it may not fully fit the definition of Classic OCD as the individual may not experience any intrusive thoughts, anxiety, or fear associated with it. They may be performing this ritual instead because of a physical sensation (premonitory urge) on their arms that only goes away once they complete the ritual. A person with Tourettic OCD may be able to suppress or delay the ritual without anxiety, whereas this wouldn't happen in a person with Classic OCD. Instead of anxiety, a person with Tourettic OCD will feel the premonitory urge getting stronger when they try to delay or stop the ritual. This can cause a rebound later on for some people or may trigger other symptoms such as rage attacks – many CBT/ERP therapists and Tourette's specialists will disagree with the last line, but this is the experience that many people with Tourette's and Tourettic OCD have reported.

Some people may find methods similar to tic redirection helpful in reducing the impact of Tourettic OCD rituals, by finding another way to satisfy the premonitory urge. CBT is unlikely to help with this as there are no thoughts or fears to talk through, and ERP may have a similar effect to tic suppression in some people. Many people with Tourettic OCD don't find the medications for Classic OCD helpful because those medications are used to reduce anxiety, but if the rituals aren't fueled by anxiety then this is unlikely to help very much. Some people with Tourettic OCD find the medications used for Tourette Syndrome helpful, such as antipsychotics as Tourettic OCD rituals are highly tic-based and fueled by premonitory sensations/urges just like tics are.

It is possible for a person to have both Tourettic OCD and Classic OCD, so care needs to be taken to differentiate what is fueling each different ritual. It is also possible for a person to grow up with T-OCD, then develop Classic OCD later, or vice versa. Despite the name, it is possible for people without TS to have Tourettic OCD as well.

Reasons For Rituals:

As explained in the previous pages, Tourettic OCD rituals occur for a different reason than Classic OCD rituals. In the graph below, I show what may fuel each ritual in Tourettic OCD vs. Classic OCD.

Ritual:	Tourettic OCD	Classic OCD
Hand Washing	Trying to wash off an uncomfortable physical sensation on the hands.	The fear of germs and getting ill.
Pulling trousers up and down when dressing	People may be trying to align an out of body sensation or knock off the feeling of a clump of energy that they sense is stuck to the clothes.	People may be afraid of their friends getting sick if they do not do the ritual, for example.
Tapping Objects	To relieve an uncomfortable sensation of an elastic band pulling you to do the ritual.	Does it as the person feels like it may neutralize negative thoughts.

OCD management:

For classic OCD, the gold-standard intervention is Cognitive Behavioral Therapy with Exposure and Response Prevention (CBT/ERP.) This is said to be effective for 75-80% of people with OCD, however, if someone doesn't respond well to it then that doesn't mean that they "aren't trying hard enough." It likely means that there's something else going on such as Tourettic OCD which needs to be managed more like tics, or PANDAS/PANS. People with PANDAS/PANS often can't respond well to psychological therapy unless the inflammation and autoimmunity is addressed first.

Medication for OCD often involves anxiety-reducing antidepressant medications such as Selective Serotonin Reuptake Inhibitors.

Acceptance and Commitment Therapy is another psychotherapy option for people with OCD. This therapy focuses on accepting the thoughts and feelings as they come without judging them, and encouraging a person to move forwards in life and stop waiting for everything to be perfect. ACT is all about accepting the present and doing what you can with what you have.

In very severe cases that don't respond well to other interventions, Transcranial Magnetic Stimulation or even Deep Brain Stimulation can be used in the management of Obsessive Compulsive Disorder.

If the OCD is caused by PANDAS/PANS, it will need to be

managed using antibiotics, anti-inflammatories, and immunomodulatory interventions to address underlying infections and reduce inflammation in the brain.

Some people report that nutritional changes can impact the severity of their OCD and work well for them. This comes under nutritional psychiatry - reducing inflammation, balancing neurotransmitters, and giving the brain the nutrients it needs to function through diet and supplements.

Bad times don't last forever, there can be a light at the end of the tunnel. Many people have been through an absolute waking nightmare only to come out of the other side and thrive.

Chapter Seven

PANDAS AND PANS

I have decided to include a chapter on PANDAS and PANS in this book, because questions about these conditions often arise in the Tourette Syndrome community due to similarities between the conditions. PANDAS and PANS can get misdiagnosed as Tourette syndrome, and it is also possible to have both TS and PANDAS/PANS, exacerbating the severity of the tics and co-occurring conditions.

PANDAS and PANS:

PANDAS stands for Paediatric Acute Onset Neuropsychiatric Disorder Associated With Streptococcal Infections. It's when a person is infected with Strep A and the immune system gets confused. In PANDAS, the immune system starts attacking part of the brain called the Basal Ganglia. This leads to symptoms such as tics, OCD, anxiety, depression, food restriction, psychosis and more. It presents differently for different people. To be diagnosed, a person will usually need to have tics or OCD.

PANS stands for Paediatric Acute Onset Neuropsychiatric Syndrome. It has the same symptoms as PANDAS, but is triggered by factors other than Strep A. PANS has both infectious and non-infectious triggers. Infectious triggers include Mycoplasma, Lyme Disease, Chickenpox, Bartonella, EBV, Influenza and pretty much any infection. Non-infectious triggers can include endocrine and metabolic issues. You need either OCD or severe food restriction plus symptoms from at least two other categories to meet PANS criteria.

A List Of Possible PANS/PANDAS Symptoms Is As Follows:

- Tics (Motor and / or vocal)
- Obsessive Compulsive Disorder
- ADHD-like traits
- Sensory processing changes
- Handwriting decline
- A decline in math ability
- Separation anxiety
- Psychosis
- Generalized anxiety
- Depression
- Mania
- Panic attacks
- Mood swings
- Dystonic symptoms
- Seizures
- Paralysis episodes
- Fatigue
- Reduced muscle tone
- Selective mutism
- Loss of the ability to speak
- Rage attacks
- Oppositional defiance
- Personality changes
- Irritability
- Insomnia
- REM behavior disorder
- Nightmares
- Delayed Sleep Phase Syndrome
- Developmental Regression

- Baby Talk
- Increased Urinary Frequency
- Urinary Incontinence
- Dilated Pupils
- Brain Fog
- Depersonalization
- Derealization
- Avoidant Restrictive Food Intake Disorder
- Symptoms that resemble Anorexia Nervosa
- Body image issues
- Swallowing issues

Not everyone has every symptom, and symptoms can change over time. Old symptoms may pass and new ones can start up in each flare.

Rages, depersonalization, and derealisation as well as pain in the shins and soles of the feet can be indicative of a Bartonella infection which can be associated with the development of PANS.

What Are The Differences Between PANDAS/PANS and Tourette Syndrome?

- Everyone with Tourette Syndrome has tics, but it is possible to have PANDAS or PANS without tics. Around 70% of people with PANDAS/PANS have tics. (Murphy et al. 2015)

- PANDAS/PANS can lead to a dramatic mental status change and can have an overnight onset (though not always) but this isn't typical of Tourette's.

- The symptoms of PANS/PANDAS can change in each flare, whereas if a person with Tourette's has tics, OCD and ADHD, they will usually stick with having that. A person with PANDAS/PANS may appear to experience tics, OCD and restrictive eating traits in their first flare, but a future flare may present with psychosis, ADHD traits, tics, derealisation, and depression instead.

- The symptoms of PANDAS/PANS will often flare dramatically with infections, whereas Tourette Syndrome symptoms often will not.

- The onset of PANDAS/PANS is more likely to occur with an infection.

- Many people with PANS/PANDAS will have symptoms such as dilated pupils, developmental regression, math decline, brain fog, seizures and a sudden personality change which are not associated with TS.

- The co-occurring conditions in people with Tourette's will often be present early on in life (such as ADHD) or will develop slowly at various stages throughout life (anxiety, depression, etc.) In contrast, PANDAS/PANS symptoms may explode and develop suddenly during a flare, looking like a person has just developed nine conditions overnight, for example.

PANDAS/PANS Is Often Misdiagnosed:

Many doctors have never heard of PANS/PANDAS, or will have been convinced by the false past narrative that it is "controversial" or "purely theoretical" despite the fact that PANDAS is recognized by the World Health Organization and PANS is recognized by both Harvard and Stanford.

Common Misdiagnoses Which People With PANDAS/PANS Often Receive Include:

- Tourette Syndrome
- Functional Neurological Disorder
- Autism
- ADHD
- Schizophrenia
- ARFID
- Bipolar Disorder
- Anxiety
- Depression
- Borderline Personality Disorder
- Dyscalculia
- Depersonalisation and Derealisation Disorder

How does one get assessed for PANDAS/PANS?

- Most doctors will just test for Strep, and if it comes back negative, they will assume the person cannot have PANDAS. This is inaccurate because a throat swab will not detect Step bacteria in areas of the body other than the throat, like a skin infection. As well as this, an ASO titre test can only detect a recent Strep infection, this is unlikely to be helpful if a person's onset was a long time ago. Seeing as PANS is triggered by infections other than Strep, it can be helpful for people to be tested for other infections such as Lyme, Mycoplasma, Bartonella, etc.

- Most doctors will assume that if a person doesn't see improvement with a week of antibiotics, they cannot have PANDAS or PANS. This is not accurate. Some people won't respond to the first antibiotic given, and will need a different type as different antibiotics target different infections. As well as this, some people are so severely affected that antibiotics on their own aren't enough. Some people need other interventions in order to see some improvement. PANS can also be triggered by viral and fungal infections, which cannot be eliminated with antibiotics. It is also possible that some people may have more complex infections with an element of antibiotic resistance such as round-body form Lyme. Some people's symptoms may be triggered by another condition such as Mast Cell Activation Syndrome, and in these cases, symptoms won't reduce until mast cells are stabilized and histamine is reduced.

- Many doctors feel uncomfortable diagnosing PANDAS and PANS, because of the outdated notion that the conditions are controversial. This is why seeing a PANDAS/PANS specialist (often in the private sector) can be best as they will know how to diagnose and treat it best.

- It is important to know that PANS is a clinical diagnosis, meaning it is diagnosed based on symptoms, clinical history and response to treatment. There is no specific blood test which can 100% prove that a person has the condition. Even the tests which assess for antibodies known to attack the brain can come back with false positives and false negatives. People with PANDAS/PANS usually have normal MRI scans so this cannot be used to diagnose.

- If you suspect that yourself or your child could have PANDAS/PANS, then it can be helpful to join online PANS communities, contact PANS charities for support, and print off leaflets on the conditions to show your primary care doctor.

- It is important to be careful as some families get falsely accused of Fabricated and Induced Illness when asking about PANDAS/PANS or seeking help from a PANS specialist as many doctors don't understand the complexity of the conditions and just assume that families are lying about or exaggerating the child's difficulties when this isn't the case.

How are PANDAS and PANS treated?

- Around 80% of people with PANS have post-infectious autoimmunity and neuroinflammation (according to The Alliance To Solve PANS and Immune-Related Encephalopathies) so in these cases it is vital to use antimicrobial and anti-inflammatory interventions.

- Immune-modulating interventions such as intravenous immunoglobulin are sometimes used. Sadly, this is not widely available in the UK.

- In extremely severe cases in America, they sometimes give Plasmapheresis and Rituximab.

- Psychotropic medications can sometimes be used for people with PANDAS and PANS, but it is advised that people with these conditions are started on a lower dose because there may be more of a risk of negative reactions. That being said, these medications can help some people, but the best result will be seen when antimicrobials, anti-inflammatories, and immune-modulating interventions are added to the mix. It is important to note though that not every PANDAS/PANS symptom can be addressed with psychotropic medications - they're unlikely to do anything for handwriting decline, coordination changes, developmental regression, etc.

- Psychological therapies such as CBT/ERP may not work for people with PANDAS/PANS until the autoimmunity has been addressed.

If your symptoms get worse when you have an infection or shortly after having an infection, it may be helpful to look into PANDAS/PANS.

Chapter Eight

RAGE ATTACKS

Rage Attacks

Rage attacks are sudden, uncontrollable outbursts of extreme anger and distress, that may be accompanied with violent actions, and verbal insults.

During a Rage Attack, A Person May:

- Hit
- Kick
- Scream
- Shout
- Say things that they do not mean
- Bite
- Push
- Scratch
- Make threats
- Throw things
- Perform any other violent action

It is important to know that rage attacks are a neurological symptom, and NOT an indication that a person is "badly behaved." rage attacks do not reflect a person's true character. The kindest and most caring person could have the most aggressive rages.

Some people refer to rage attacks as neuro storms, as they are just that - neurological storms. The rage attacks are involuntary and have a neurological basis.

Rage Attacks Can Be Experienced Differently By Different People:

Although rage attacks usually are not the same as tics, they are just as involuntary as the tics. During a rage attack, a person loses control of their rational thinking and actions, and is likely to do things that they do not mean. Although the typical consensus is that rage attacks are anger-based, a small percentage of people may actually have tic rages. This is where the rage attacks ARE tics, they can be exclusively tic-based. For example, a person may have an episode of hitting, biting, scratching, throwing, and yelling tics, which may resemble an anger-based rage, but is not one. In a tic rage, a person is usually not actually angry, their tics are just making them perform violent actions uncontrollably. However, the majority of rages are anger-based, but this doesn't make them any less involuntary.

Discipline is Unlikely to Help or Prevent Rage Attacks:

Punishing a person after a rage attack is unlikely to be helpful, as it will not prevent the attacks. Rage attacks are a neurological symptom that can come in episodes, like seizures or tic attacks, therefore disciplining someone for something that is involuntary is unlikely to be helpful, and may just end up destroying a person's self-esteem.

If a person is made to feel 'naughty' or 'bad' for something that they cannot control, then this can break down someone's confidence and sense of self-worth. People feel unworthy of love as they may feel like they are a 'bad person' who is 'mean' and 'lacks self-discipline', when this is false. The person has a neurological condition which causes these outbursts that are out of the individual's control and say nothing about who they are as a person.

Rage Attacks Can Occur More In One Environment Than Another:

Some people report that they experience rage attacks more in the home environment than in the school or work environment. This does NOT indicate that there is anything wrong with the home environment, it is more likely that the person experiences more rages at home as they are holding it all in whilst in school, so that it all explodes once a person gets home. In school, a person may be afraid of being judged by their peers and teachers, or they may be afraid of being punished for a symptom. Therefore, people are more likely to let it all out once they are at home, because they love their parents and know that they will be able to support them and won't judge them.

Triggers For Rage Attacks:

Different people report different triggers for their rage attacks. Although a rage attack may appear to be triggered by something very small, that is unlikely to be the root trigger. That 'small' thing could just be what sent the person 'over the edge' when they were already distressed.

Rage Attack Triggers Can Include:

- **Food Dye Sensitivity** – Many people with Tourette Syndrome and PANS/PANDAS report that food dye consumption can lead to explosive outbursts. There is a mountain of evidence that shows how food dye consumption can trigger neurological symptoms such as hyperactivity. One example is the Southampton six study which demonstrated how mixtures of artificial dyes and sodium benzoate can trigger hyperactivity in pre-school and primary school-aged children. This study is the main reason why foods with certain artificial dyes in need to have a warning label on them in the UK stating that they can have an impact on activity and attention in children. In people who get aggressive after the consumption of certain dyes, their brain may show increased activity on a SPECT scan after they eat the dyes, as demonstrated by Amen Clinics. It isn't just red food dye that can trigger these symptoms, it is any artificial dye along with a natural dye called Annatto which many people are sensitive to. The Hyperactive Children's Support Group and The Feingold Association have information on the neurological effects of food dye consumption on their websites.

- **Tic Suppression** – Holding in tics can be extremely uncomfortable for an individual and can make symptoms worse later on. For some people, the tic urge may accumulate and become physically intolerable for some people, this could make a person appear snappy and pressured, as their body may feel as if it is filled to the brim with pressure and tension. This can then explode out as a rage attack.

- **OCD rituals not being fulfilled** – Many people with Tourette Syndrome and PANS/PANDAS have OCD, and when a ritual goes unfilled, such as when working on Exposure therapy, it may lead to an increased level of anxiety and discomfort, which can then trigger a rage attack.

- **Hidden learning difficulties** – Learning difficulties such as Dyscalculia are common in people with Tourette Syndrome, and a decline in maths ability can be a symptom of PANS/PANDAS. This could make math classes at school, or the need to do mathematics at work, incredibly frustrating and anxiety-provoking for some people. This could lead to rage attacks. As well as this, a person may judge themselves as 'not being smart' if they struggle with something like this. This could then lower someone's self-esteem and cause more frustration, therefore leading to meltdowns and rages.

- **Infections** – Particularly if a person has PANS/PANDAS, infections can trigger brain inflammation leading to rage attacks and exacerbated tics.

- **An object being moved, or things being in the 'wrong place'** – if someone has OCD or OCD traits then this can be infuriating.

- **Under Stimulation or Over Stimulation** - If a person has ADHD or sensory processing issues, then they may struggle with feelings of under-stimulation or overstimulation.

This may seem counterintuitive, but some people with ADHD traits find that they need more stimulation, in order to calm the over-activity in their body and mind. It is as if the hyperactivity is a sort of coping mechanism for feeling chronically under-stimulated. This is why some people may need something that is stimulating for them, such as listening to fast-paced music (as long as this doesn't exacerbate the tics), exercising, dancing, fidgeting, or moving around in order to feel calm. It is also possible that some people with hyperactivity will need a calmer environment, with less stimulation or excitement, as everyone is different and everyone's brain has different needs.

Sensory processing issues can lead to overstimulation or under-stimulation, depending on the way sensory information is being processed. Under-stimulation may trigger rage attacks as someone may become so antsy and irritable due to not being able to get the stimulation which their body and brain need. Over-stimulation may trigger rage attacks as people may get overwhelmed by all of the sensory input which their brain cannot process.

Rage triggers are different for different people and it is likely that different triggers are playing a role at the same time. It can take some detective work, but finding out what the triggers are and addressing them

can reduce the attacks.

How To Support Someone Having A Rage Attack:

- When the attack is happening, try to refrain from reasoning with the individual. During a rage attack, a person cannot process what you are saying to them. They cannot take it in. It will only frustrate and overwhelm them further, which could prolong the attack and make it more intense.

- Ensure that the individual is not hurting themselves.

- Once the attack has passed, reassure them that they are still a good person and that you still love them no matter what. Reassure them that you know that they cannot control their rage attacks.

- If needed, give the individual some space after the attack, as long as they are not at risk of causing any harm to themselves. Some people need a bit of personal space or alone time after a rage attack, and they may appear to 'zone out' and dissociate. If the person experiences bouts of unresponsiveness, then rule out absence seizures.

- Be kind to the person. Comfort them when the attack is over and when they are ready for contact with others. A person will often feel extremely guilty and shameful after a rage attack, so let them know that it is okay. You know it is a neurological symptom.

- Remember that a person having a rage attack likely knows that the actions they perform in the attack are not appropriate, but they cannot control it. Therefore, for a person who understands this, telling them that what they did isn't appropriate is not going to help, as they already know this.

- Take threats of suicide and self-harm seriously.

- Do not punish an individual for having a rage attack. It is possible to help them know that they can be held accountable for their actions, by allowing them to help out with fixing or replacing anything they have broken, but this can only be done if the person is well enough and if the rages aren't so frequent that things get broken all the time. Punishment shouldn't be an option as rages are an involuntary symptom.

- Try not to take what is said to others during a rage attack personally. Many people having a rage attack will say things such as "I hate you!", "You did this to me", or "I wish you were dead!" A person doesn't mean it when they say these things during a rage attack. It can be hard not to take personally, but the individual doesn't mean it.

- Stay calm. The person experiencing a rage attack needs you to be calm, soothing and caring. If you are stern or strict, the person is likely to become more anxious and this can make it worse.

- Move fragile objects away from the person so that

they do not get broken.

- Some people find distraction, humour, or calming techniques helpful, but sometimes people are too deep into the rage attack for this to work.

- Move sharp or heavy objects away so that the individual doesn't use it to harm themselves or use it as a weapon.

- Never make threats like "If you do this again we will take away your TV." This is likely to make a person more anxious and is very unlikely to reduce the rage attacks as they are an uncontrollable symptom which the person doesn't want to experience.

- After a rage attack, let the person rest. They are likely exhausted.

How To Prevent Rage Attacks:

- Avoid triggers, look into potential dietary triggers.

- Remind the person to set boundaries, take things easy, and look after themselves. Reducing stress may be beneficial.

- Some people may find it helpful to learn calming techniques or ways to redirect rages, but this may not have any beneficial effect for some people.

- Reduce or stop tic suppression, this does not mean

stopping tic management strategies, it means not to forcefully hold tics in.

- Seek the help of a professional for interventions such as medication that may reduce rages. Don't be afraid to consider natural options as well though as a functional medicine doctor, naturopath, or nutritional therapist may help you find some underlying biochemical triggers.

- If you have PANS/PANDAS, reduce the likelihood of going into a flare by practicing reasonable infection avoidance techniques, such as requiring that Strep cases are reported in school, and any surface which the student with Strep or another triggering infection has touched must be decontaminated to avoid the student with PANS/PANDAS from coming into contact with the pathogen.

- See what the individual's sensory needs are, and meet them. Encourage the use of sensory aids such as sunglasses and ear defenders. People with neurological issues do not have a problem with anxiety causing their sensory processing issues, they have a neurological difference meaning that their brain cannot process sensory information in the correct way, which can sometimes be mistaken for anxiety. Due to this, exposure therapy which is normally used for anxiety disorders will not work in reducing sensory processing issues as the person will just learn to dissociate in order to not feel the anxiety around the sensory input, but the sensitivity is still there causing other issues such as increased tics, headaches, meltdowns, and hyperactivity. No amount of exposure will change the physical and genetic differences that caused the sensory processing issues, so exposure will only teach the person that they should stay in environments that make them uncomfortable and make their symptoms worse. This is not the message we want to be sending. Encouraging the person to use sensory aids will reduce symptoms that are triggered by and exacerbated by sensory input, and teach the person that they don't have to tolerate discomfort if it is harming them.

- Ensure that the person is getting the appropriate accommodations in school and in the workplace.

Coming into contact with doctors who don't understand rage attacks:

Most doctors don't understand rage attacks - this includes Tourette's specialists and mental health specialists. They will usually tell you that the individual is doing them intentionally and that they are just badly behaved. This is a form of medical gaslighting. This type of attitude from medical personnel leads to the individual developing low self-esteem and trauma responses from being blamed for, and punished for, a symptom that is out of their control.

Parents are sadly often blamed as well, and told they are bad parents who need to do a better job. This is not true, rages are neurological and have nothing to do with parenting. Tourette's is a genetic condition and rages are a fairly common symptom. This is not your fault, or your child's fault. You may get sent to a parenting course, but these courses are rarely, if ever, tailored to the needs of young people with Tourette's or PANDAS/PANS, and are virtually never made with the input of Tourettic individuals. This is why you have to take these courses with a grain of salt, as no one understands your child like you do. Always believe your child over the doctors and therapists.

Facts About Rage Attacks:

- Rage Attacks can be tic-based or anger-based, both are uncontrollable.

- Rage Attacks are fairly common symptoms of Tourette Syndrome and PANS/PANDAS.

- Rage Attacks are neither the fault of the individual nor the parents of the individual.

- Rage Attacks are NOT bad behavior, they are a neurological symptom. Rages do NOT reflect a person's personality. A person likely knows that what they do in a rage attack is inappropriate, but they are NOT choosing to do it.

Consequences of being punished for rage attacks and related symptoms:

Being punished for an involuntary symptom like rages or tics is the same as being punished for blinking or breathing. A person doesn't choose to experience these symptoms. If a person is punished for their symptoms, it can cause long-term trauma responses, such as:

- Low self-esteem.
- Self-blame.
- The inner belief of being "evil" in some way.
- Over defensiveness.
- Fears around going to the doctors in case they get blamed for their symptoms.
- Self-punishment such as self-harm, as the individual has been taught that they deserve to be punished for struggling.
- Increased masking of neurodivergent traits.
- Feeling the need to over-explain symptoms so that people don't judge you.
- Suicidal thoughts.
- Intense guilt and remorse for experiencing uncontrollable symptoms.
- Dissociation related to the fear of showing emotion, in case it leads to punishment.
- Flashbacks related to being punished or harmfully restrained for symptoms.
- Excessive people-pleasing traits due to the fear of being seen as a bad person for experiencing symptoms.

Rage attacks do not make you a bad person. They are a symptom in the same way that tics are a symptom.

Chapter Nine

TOURETTE'S THROUGHOUT THE LIFESPAN

Tics Throughout The Lifespan

Tourette Syndrome is a lifelong condition, but it may impact you differently depending on what stage of your life you are in.

People are born with the genetic predisposition to develop TS, but they are not born ticcing. Tics usually develop during early childhood, around the age of 7. However, some people don't experience noticeable symptoms until their teenage years.

Tourette Syndrome in the early years - Ages 3-9:
During this time in a person's life, they will be settling into school life. It is important for the school to be made aware of any difficulties that the child has so that they can put the appropriate support in place. Support in school will not stop the tics, but it will reduce an individual's stress and will allow them to get the most out of school life. ADHD symptoms are likely to be noticed around this age, and tics often start around this time as well.

In Tourette Syndrome, tics often start in the face, neck, and shoulders, though some people do have more complex tics to begin with. A child may be confused as to why they are experiencing these urges, uncontrollable movements, and vocalizations. A child's diagnosis should never be hidden from them. It isn't disempowering for a child to know that they have a disability, it is more disempowering for them to not know and to incorrectly judge themselves as "weak", "weird", or "lacking willpower". Being aware of their condition can allow the child to understand themselves instead of judge themselves. During this phase of childhood, children usually have one specific class teacher so it is easier to create consistency in regard to accommodations and support given in school as it is usually only the class teacher who needs to be aware of the support that is needed.

The pre-pubertal years - **Ages 10-12:** During this time, a child is preparing to move to middle/secondary school, and then will be moving to the new school. Many people see an increase in tics around this time for a variety of reasons. One of the main reasons why tics can get worse around this time is because the transition from elementary school to middle/secondary school is a big one. Suddenly, instead of just having one teacher, the student has a different teacher for every subject and has to move between classes each lesson. This can increase anxiety and therefore worsen tics. As mentioned before, many people with Tourette Syndrome have sensory processing issues, which can make middle/secondary school challenging as it is much more crowded than elementary school. This can be overwhelming for some people.

In secondary/middle school, the student will likely have a mix of different teachers. Some of their new teachers will be understanding of Tourette Syndrome, while others may not be. It is vital that a student is told how to advocate for themselves and explain their condition around this age so that they don't get discriminated against or punished for something that they cannot control. Some people find it helpful to print out information leaflets for teachers who do not understand. It is also important to make sure that meetings with the SENCO are made prior to the student starting the school to make sure they know how to meet the child's needs. If this is not possible, then it is important to have a meeting with the Special Educational Needs Coordinator shortly after the child starts at the new school. It is vital to educate the school on how Tourette's is not a behavioral problem, but is a neurological condition, and how it is not possible to discipline tics out of a person.

Some young people may actually benefit from the change in environment from elementary to middle school as it may allow them to let go of unhealthy habits such as tic suppression. Being in a new environment may allow them to stop holding in tics as much, as it is a new start. Suppressing tics less may allow a person to focus better and may reduce the incidence of tic explosions when arriving home.

The teenage years - ages 13-17: The teenage years are hard for anyone, but when you are dealing with neurological and psychiatric differences like Tourette Syndrome, ADHD, OCD, and more on top of that - it can be a nightmare. That being said, young people have usually settled into high school by this time and may have a list of accommodations that are in place. Accommodations may need to be changed over time depending on how someone is impacted by their conditions.

Some people find that hormonal changes, such as those

associated with periods, can cause tics to flare up. As well as this, young people may become more interested in romantic relationships during this time which may cause extra anxiety as the young person may worry about potential romantic partners judging them due to their tics.

Schools tend to put a lot of pressure on teenagers, especially as it gets closer to their final exams. Many people with Tourette Syndrome find that their tics get worse around this time due to stress. It is essential for teenagers to know that regardless of how they do in their exams, they should still be proud of themselves because just going to school when you have TS can be daunting and should therefore be celebrated regardless of what exam results a person gets.

It is absolutely vital that exam arrangements are put in place for the individual so that they get the same chance of success as anyone else. Most people with Tourette Syndrome will need a separate room for exams so that they don't worry about distracting others with their tics. Many young people also find it helpful to have extra time and rest breaks so that if they have a bad episode of tics during an exam, it doesn't eat up their exam time.

Do not let the school make excuses and say that they cannot provide access arrangements, because they have to make reasonable adjustments. If a student is anxious that their access arrangements may not be put in place, they may not feel able to attend school on the day of the exam. The young person must be taught to advocate for themselves and to not take no as an answer when it comes to accommodations. Accommodations and adjustments are a necessity for someone with such a complex condition, not a luxury.

The early adult years - **18-25:** Many people are told that they will grow out of their Tourette's symptoms once they reach adulthood, but the symptoms don't magically disappear at the age of 18. Some people do find that their tics get much milder during the adult years, but this doesn't always happen. Being an adult with Tourette's brings new challenges. Some people are happy to leave the school environment, whilst others struggle without the support network of having school staff and peers around them.

Some people with TS go to university, and others go down other avenues. Whatever someone chooses to do, it is valid. Suppose the individual does end up going to university - in that case, it can be a big jump from living with parents in the family home, to moving into student accommodation and learning how to be independent.

Being in university can allow the individual to become more confident in terms of advocating for themselves, because the responsibility for requesting the support needed in university is placed more on the individual than on their parents.

University life can give the person a new opportunity to make friends with people who understand them and who will root for them. By the time people are in university, people have usually matured enough not to make fun of someone for being different, so it may be easier to find friends who are accepting.

In university, the individual will have to find out what study methods work best for them, and those methods will likely be different from the ones their neurotypical peers find helpful. A Tourettic individual has to work with their unique neurology, not against it. The chapter titled "Coping with Tourette's in school" contains some study tips which may be helpful for Tourettic university students as well as school students.

During the young adult years, many people will be navigating work life, and figuring out how and when to let their employer know about their condition. Some people prefer not to tell an employer that they have TS until they have secured a job through writing, because if you tell them afterwards and they discriminate against you, it is easier to take legal action. There are some instances however where a person isn't able to suppress their tics and where their tics are incredibly noticeable - it may not be possible to hide them during an interview, so some people do need to disclose it straight away.

Some people like to frame their condition in a positive light to employers, by saying how it helps them be more empathetic, insightful, energetic, etc. It can be helpful to highlight the strengths to an employer if you do disclose it to them so that they don't just make negative assumptions.

During these years, people often try to get into romantic relationships. It is vital to have a partner who is accepting of Tourette Syndrome, and who isn't bothered or offended by the tics.

Red flags in a relationship as a Tourettic person include:

- Your partner telling you that you would be better without tics.
- Your partner constantly tells you how much your tics are bothering them.
- Your partner pressuring you to suppress tics.
- Your partner telling you to tic quietly.
- Your partner making you feel like an inconvenience for having tics, OCD, ADHD, etc.

If your partner keeps saying or doing these things after you have told them how it makes you feel, they are likely not the best person for you to be with as it is unhealthy for you to be in a relationship like that.

Ages 25-50: During this time, people may or may not be thinking about having children. Tourette Syndrome will usually not impact an individual's ability to parent - most people with TS can make great parents!

Some people who are considering having children may be worried about passing Tourette's onto their child as the condition is genetic and tends to run in families. People need to know that even if their child does have TS, then they will be the best parents for that child as they know exactly how it feels and will be able to support them well. Some people choose not to have kids as they are afraid that their children will struggle in the same way they have. That is also a valid way to feel.

At this age, those who are able to work will have likely settled into working life - but sadly this doesn't mean that the struggles are over. People may still face discrimination, have to repeatedly advocate for their needs, or struggle with employment gaps. Some people however thrive once they are in an accepting environment, so for people in a long-term work placement, things may become easier for them as they know they're in an environment that accepts them and knows their needs.

People around this age may find that there's less support available than when they were a child. Most TS specialists and events are geared towards children and young people with the condition - so it can be difficult to navigate adulthood with the condition.

Some people find that co-occurring ADHD symptoms can get milder as they get older, but not everyone experiences this.

Many adults with Tourette Syndrome have no problem living independently, others need the support of carers to perform daily tasks and keep them safe and may need extra support such as an assistance dog or home accommodations.

Do be aware that there are some people who don't even get diagnosed with Tourette's until adulthood, as their symptoms may have been brushed off in childhood and only become more noticeable in adult life.

As the individual starts getting older, the repetitive movements may start taking more of a toll on the individual's body. People may start experiencing more pain and general wear and tear from decades of constant movement. Thankfully, many people find pain relief options to help manage this.

In women, tics are less likely to reduce with age and may be more physically disabling in adulthood. (Garris, 2021) As people get older, they may develop more co-occurring mental health difficulties such as anxiety and depression - though this thankfully isn't always the case. Migraines also appear to occur frequently in Tourettic people, (Kwack, 2003) so these may emerge in adulthood for some people if they don't develop them in childhood.

Joint hypermobility is more common in people with Tourette Syndrome than in the general population, just like how many Autistic people have joint hypermobility syndromes as well. For some people, pain and joint instability related to hypermobility may start to cause more problems in adulthood.

Age 50 plus: Some people's tics mellow when they're older. Many people find that ADHD traits also reduce as they get older - however, women often find that their ADHD traits get worse during perimenopause or menopause as the hormone changes can alter the level of neurotransmitters in the brain.

The physical toll of having tics may start to show more at this age, as the decades' worth of repetitive movements may have caused wear and tear to the joints and may have caused people to develop trapped or compressed nerves from the complex movements. However, this isn't the case for everyone as some people's tics do decrease with age and aren't frequent enough to cause these types of issues. Do be aware that this wear and tear can actually become noticeable as early as in a person's early 20s, but when the individual is over 50 years old it is likely to be even more noticeable.

I do want to note however, that even if an individual's tics don't decrease with age, things can still get easier as people may come to accept themselves more as they get older and find management strategies that truly work for them.

This is just an example of how TS and related conditions may present throughout a person's life. Everyone is different and not everyone has co-occurring conditions such as ADHD or Migraines.

Chapter Ten

COPING WITH TOURETTE'S IN SCHOOL

School Accommodations For Tourette's and Related Conditions

Having support in school is vital for people with Tourette's and related conditions because without it they may struggle to get through school at all. Having this support put in place can allow the student to feel at ease in an inclusive school environment. Schools have the duty to provide reasonable adjustments and make accommodations to meet the student's needs.

One of the most important things when working with a pupil who has Tourette Syndrome or a related condition is to not punish the symptoms as they are neurological and involuntary. This includes the tics, OCD compulsions, rage attacks and ADHD traits. Instead, it is more important to understand and accept the student whilst helping the student in a way that works for them.

A list of possible accommodations is as follows, it is important to remember that this is not a complete list as support will have to be tailored to the individual. These are just some ideas of support that could be put in place.

- **A time-out card** - A time-out card can allow the Tourettic person to go and take a short break out of the classroom in order to let off some steam, cool off, use coping mechanisms or regulate emotions. Some people may be able to leave the classroom to go and work in a separate room if their tics, OCD or anxiety are too severe for the pupil to function in the classroom. It is important to note that an individual should never be told to leave the classroom as that could be classed as discrimination, but an individual can choose to leave the class if they think that it would be beneficial to their wellbeing or if they can feel some severe tics coming on and would rather be in another setting.

- **Half days or a reduced timetable** – Some people with Tourette's will need half days or a reduced timetable in order to reduce anxiety and decrease the amount of time ticcing if tics are worse in the school environment due to sensory stimulation.

- **Skip the lunch queue** – Some young people with ADHD may need to skip the lunch queue if they cannot wait in line due to hyperactivity and some people may need to skip the queue if they have tics that include hitting out, kicking or full body movements so that they don't accidentally touch someone in the queue.

- **A reminder card** – Some people may need a card on a lanyard or keychain that reminds them not to forget certain things such as their homework or PE kit, as some people may walk out of classes without essential items or possessions. They may lose things if they struggle with executive dysfunction or ADHD symptoms. It is also important that teachers are understanding if a student doesn't have the necessary equipment or forgets things as the person doesn't want to forget things. They want to be organized but their brain won't let them.

- **Have a mentor** - Some people have a mentor who they can go and speak to if they are struggling. A mentor can also sometimes help someone work through any emotional issues or worries that may arise in the school environment. They can also sometimes help people manage their workload. A mentor could be a trusted member of staff or even an older student who volunteers to help younger students in the school setting.

- **Homework extensions and exemptions:** When dealing with Tourette's, OCD, ADHD, Depression, and any other issues that an individual may be facing, it can be exceedingly difficult to complete homework on time, if at all. OCD may mean that hours of an individual's day is taken up by debilitating rituals that leave them with no time to do the homework, or their intrusive thoughts and anxiety may be so severe that they are exhausted once they return home and need to rest. For some people, they may have been harmfully suppressing tics in the school environment, leading to rebounds and explosions of severe symptoms when they get home, meaning they are unable to complete the homework. Conversely, they may be exhausted from ticcing all day in school so they might need to use their time at home to relax. Some people with ADHD may struggle with executive dysfunction and time sense issues, where they procrastinate doing the work until the last minute, so they may need an extension. This is a neurological issue and not a choice. The individual literally has a skewed sense of time. For some people, co-occurring mental health issues such as Depression can lead to emotional distress and a lack of motivation. This can make getting work done difficult and a person's mental well-being is always more important than their grades. One thing I would say to people with Tourette's and related conditions reading this is that it is okay to ask for help and to ask for extensions. Sometimes we tend to judge ourselves and think that we are not trying hard enough, but in fact, we are working so much harder than most people as we are trying to do the work with a brain that doesn't always want to cooperate. Therefore, the homework extensions and exemptions are a reasonable adjustment.

- **Modifications to how work is done by the individual in lessons** - Sometimes tics and other symptoms can make it difficult to do certain tasks in the same way as the other students. For example, a student's OCD may be so severe that it causes them to take a long time to dress themselves. This could make dressing for gym lessons extremely challenging, so instead of changing into their kit, a person may be given permission to just take off their tie and put on some trainers and do lessons like that. Different modifications will be needed for different people as we all have different needs so it does have to be tailored to the individual. Being able to work around the tics and other symptoms by changing the way some activities are done can be helpful as an individual can be given a chance to succeed by doing something in their own way.

- **Tuition** - Tourette syndrome doesn't affect intelligence, however, some people may have co-occurring specific learning difficulties such as Dyscalculia, which is a difficulty with maths / mental arithmetic, so an individual may need extra support or tuition to ensure that they are making progress in those classes. Some people may have more severe tics in some classes meaning that they struggle to focus and retain information, so having tuition sessions could allow them to go over what has been taught in class, and if people are out of class a lot because of the symptoms then tuition can ensure that they are catching up and not behind on their work.

- **Some people may prefer to do work in a smaller group or separately out of the classroom** if they think that it would benefit them and help them learn - this has to be an individual's choice, they cannot be sent out of class as this could be seen as discrimination.

- **Being allowed to chew gum in class** - Some people find that chewing gum can help reduce vocal tics. It doesn't stop them as it's not a cure, but can help someone manage and redirect tics so that they do not become disruptive to the individual's learning. Chewing gum should not be used if there is any risk of choking or if people have breathing tics where they may inhale the gum.

- **Permission to use fidget tools** - Some people find that fidgeting can reduce restlessness and therefore decrease their tics. Fidget tools are also incredibly useful for people with ADHD as physically moving the hands around can slow someone's mind down and can allow them to focus. Some people also find that fidgeting helps to reduce feelings of nervousness and anxiety.

- **Leaving classes early** - Some people find it beneficial to leave class 5 minutes early to avoid being near too many other people in the corridors in between classes and to avoid excess sensory input which may worsen tics and anxiety. Some people may leave class up to 15 minutes early to have a break from class, to relax before the next lesson starts and to let more tics out to avoid suppression.

- **Having lunch in a smaller setting** - Some people can be overwhelmed by all of the stimulation in the lunch hall, and this sensory input can make tics worse. As well as this, being near so many people can trigger anxiety. Having lunch in a smaller setting or with a small group of friends can sometimes be arranged.

- **Missing assemblies** - Some people might have to miss assemblies because they may be too anxious to attend. Imagine sitting in a quiet room packed with lots of people, and having a condition that makes it difficult not to draw attention to yourself as you involuntarily make noises. This is why people can be given permission not to attend assemblies if they find it too difficult. Nobody should ever be encouraged to suppress symptoms so it is important to work around it and allow someone to leave if they do not feel comfortable in the assembly hall. It is important, however, not to send people out or tell them that they have to leave as this would be discrimination. It has to be the individual's choice.

- **Having a laptop/word processor in class and in exams** - Some tics can make it difficult to write as they may make the person throw pens, rip up paper, scribble over the page, or have hand tics or writing tics such as coprographia which make it difficult to complete written work. Some people also have co-occurring Dysgraphia or hypermobility which can make it difficult to write, so having a laptop to take notes and do work on can be beneficial. However, this may not work for everyone as some people may have compulsions where they repeatedly delete and retype words or keep scrolling up and down the page a certain number of times. Some people may have tics such as hitting or smashing the laptop which can be harmful. In these cases, a person may find it helpful to have a scribe, where they say what they want to write and a teaching assistant writes it down for them.

- **Using other people's notes** - If the student is struggling to write or focus in class, then the teacher could photocopy another classmate's notes with their permission and share it with the individual.

- **Skip reading out loud** - Some people may become

very anxious at the thought of reading out loud in front of the class and they might have OCD rituals where they read the same line repeatedly. A person's vocal tics may become more prominent when reading aloud so it is important to allow the individual to skip reading out loud if it might make them self-conscious or if it is too difficult for them.

- **Laminated sheets** - Having laminated worksheets can be beneficial if an individual has tics that involve ripping up paper, and then they can write on it using a whiteboard pen or a permanent marker.

- **Have seating arrangements where people are not near any distractions and can leave class easily** if they feel something coming on like an episode of severe tics or anxiety.

- **Audiobooks** - These can be helpful if people have OCD rituals that involve rereading lines or if people have tics that make it difficult to read such as blinking or ripping out the pages, and some people with ADHD may find it easier to focus on an audiobook than on reading text.

- **Be understanding of poor presentation and poor handwriting** - Many people in the Tourette's community have difficulties with handwriting and presentation due to hand tics, OCD causing them to go over certain letters when writing, dysgraphia, hypermobility, visual processing issues and undetected PANS/PANDAS. It is important not to punish someone for their handwriting or presentation difficulties as the person does want to do their work neatly, but it can be virtually impossible sometimes due to symptoms.

- **Keep the desks as clear as possible** - This is because some people may get easily distracted but also because some students may have tics that involve throwing items across the classroom.

- **A social and emotional group** - Some schools have social and emotional groups where the students can talk about their emotions and develop social skills. It can help people cope with and manage difficult emotions and can allow people to make friends. Social groups should NEVER encourage tic suppression or try to teach someone why their symptoms are "socially unacceptable" because symptoms associated with Tourette Syndrome are involuntary.

- **Allow the student to move around as they do their work** - A lot of people with Tourette's have ADHD or ADHD-like traits and that can make it virtually impossible to stay still. It is important to let someone stand up, move around, and fidget so that they can feel at ease and focus in class. It is important for people to understand that the student may work in a different way to others, but that shouldn't be an issue as it is what works for them.

- **Provide activity breaks** - Some people cannot sit still for long periods of time so some teachers may incorporate a mini dance break into the middle of the class to keep students focused and stimulated.

- **Having class notes emailed to the individual or put onto an online portal after class** - Tics, OCD and ADHD can make it difficult to get all of the information down and focus so having the notes available after class can be beneficial.

- **Extra time in exams** - Some people need extra time in exams as the tics, intrusive thoughts and ADHD traits can make it very difficult to focus or write all of the answers down. Having extra time can also relieve some tension and anxiety so that people can have a clearer mind when completing the paper, and the anxiety reduction can also lead to a reduction in tics. Most people have 25% extra time, but some people have 100% extra time so the pupil does not need to rush and so that people with near-constant tics get a fair chance.

- **Rest breaks for exams** - Some people may need rest breaks during exams where they can stop and have a break whilst being supervised by the invigilator. This can be beneficial in terms of reducing anxiety and allowing people to regain focus. It is also helpful as people can "stop the clock" if they have a tic attack and then go back to the test once the attack is over without losing any exam time.

- **Having a separate room for exams** - Some people have a separate room for exams with just the individual and the invigilator, this is beneficial as the student can tic freely without worrying about disturbing others and it can also reduce general anxiety.

Teachers need to be understanding and empathetic towards the challenges a student may be facing. There are many other issues that students with Tourette's might face in the school environment aside from the tics as many symptoms are hidden such as intrusive thoughts, mental tics, inattention, executive dysfunction, anxiety, strong premonitory urges and more.

How Do I Get My Teachers To Understand My Tics?

Educating your teachers on your tics is extremely important because if they understand what is going on, they are going to be more equipped to support you in school and they are less likely to be discriminatory towards you or manage your tics in an inappropriate way. It is never your fault if a teacher sends you out of the class or discriminates against you in some way due to ticcing, but sometimes if they are more aware of what is going on it may be less likely to happen, but if it does then you know that they are doing it whilst knowing that they shouldn't, so that's even worse.

Ways To Educate Teachers About Tics:

1) **At the beginning of the school year, you could email your teachers and explain that you have tics.** You could say what helps and what doesn't help, and you could explain that your tics are unintentional, not a

reflection of your character, and that they are not within your control. You could outline the kind of support that you will need in class and say that you will enjoy spending the next academic year with them. If you do not have the teacher's email addresses, or if you feel they may not listen, then you could ask the Special Educational Needs Coordinator to contact all of your teachers to inform them of your condition.

2) **You could type up a letter about your tics** and include information on how you would like teachers to react, and what teachers shouldn't do, and then put it in your pencil case. If you come across a substitute/cover teacher who may be unaware of your condition, then you could show them the letter before the class starts so they understand your tics, or you could show the letter to a teacher who is reacting to your tics in an unhelpful way so that they can understand more and stop reacting in an unhelpful manner.

3) **Give your teachers a leaflet.** Some Tourette's organizations have leaflets on the conditions. Please make sure that the leaflet is accurate and does NOT advocate for tic suppression. Giving your teachers a leaflet gives them a chance to understand your condition and learn how to support you best.

4) **Challenge discrimination as soon as possible.** You never deserve to be discriminated against or treated badly due to your tics or anything else. It is important to report discrimination as soon as you can to prevent it from happening again.

You could report an incident of this manner by talking to the Special Educational Needs Coordinator, who may be able to educate the teacher who is responsible. You could also report it to the headteacher, and get your parents to make a formal complaint. If they are not doing anything about the situation, then threaten to report the school's negligence to the school's inspection and education authority.

If a teacher is aware that you have tics, they should not be allowed to get away with:

- Sending you out of class for ticcing. This is akin to sending a student out for being in a wheelchair.
- Telling you to stop ticcing, or to tic quietly.
- Making nasty comments towards you.
- Refusing to accommodate your needs by not giving you adjustments. The Equality Act 2010 states that reasonable adjustments must be made. This is a piece of legislation in the United Kingdom.
- Punishing you for ticcing.

Please report any instances of these occurring to a member of staff who has the capacity to deal with these concerns, situations, and complaints. You deserve better. Never purposefully insult a teacher for reacting to your tics in an unhelpful manner, as this makes the situation worse. Instead, stick up for yourself in a formal manner by saying "I have tics, they are an involuntary symptom. By doing this, you are discriminating against me on the basis of me having a disability. My tics are unintentional and I do not mean what I tic, they are misfired signals from my brain and they are not a reflection of my character." Sticking up for yourself and educating others is important, for it could prevent another person with tics from facing the same discrimination from that teacher or member of staff.

How Do I Educate My Classmates?

It can be helpful to educate your classmates about your tics so that they know what is going on and so that you can help create a more understanding and accepting generation. Sometimes, if classmates understand your condition then they may be less likely to be unkind about your tics. However, educating them may not completely stop negative reactions, but it may reduce some of them if people are given the opportunity to understand.

Here are some ideas on ways to educate classmates about your Tourette's:

1. **Do a whole school or whole year group assembly.** This can be daunting, but very helpful. If you have tics which are loud, complex, and very noticeable in corridors then it can be helpful to inform the whole school about what is going on when they see you tic. You could make a presentation or video and show it in the assembly. You could be brave and present it yourself or a teacher or advocate could do it for you or alongside you.

I recommend showing examples of how serious tics can be. You want to get the facts across, but you also want to get to people's emotional sides as that is what may make them realize that they shouldn't be teasing you for ticcing or seeing it all as a big joke. If people are able to see how distressing and disabling it can be to have tics then they may feel more guilt and remorse if they tease you for it and people may have more empathy, compassion and understanding towards you.

2. **Do a class presentation.** If you find it too daunting or if you feel it is unnecessary to do a whole school assembly, then you could do a mini-class presentation just to make people in your class aware of why you make movements and sounds you cannot control.

3. **Do not let people get away with bullying you.** You deserve better, and they need to be educated. Report any instances of bullying to a member of staff.

Tips For Studying And Doing Assignments When You're Neurodivergent:

1. Work smart, not just hard: This isn't to discourage people from working hard. However, because so many people with Tourette's struggle with inattention, it can be helpful to have shorter revision sessions that focus on the main point, rather than long ones that cover everything. The mind probably isn't going to be able to pay attention to everything and may miss important information otherwise. For example, rather than reading through an entire novel for English class, it may be helpful for someone to go on a website that allows them to memorize individual quotes and get a summary of the overall story. This will be more helpful for a person with inattention than reading a whole book, as they may zone out when reading the book, but the shortened quotes will stick out to them more.

2. **Make use of the accessibility features on technology:** Some phones, laptops, and computers have a feature where you can highlight text and it will read it out to you. This can be helpful for people with reading comprehension problems and for people who struggle to take in what they are reading due to inattention and hyperactivity. Speech-to-text may also be helpful for people who struggle to type due to motor tics or severe hyperactivity meaning that typing one letter at a time makes them incredibly restless and uncomfortable.

3. **Let yourself move around:** Sometimes, the only way to slow your mind down when you have hyperactivity is to let your body move around so that you can let the hyperactivity out in another way. Physically moving around may also release some of the uncomfortable premonitory sensations associated with having tics. Don't be afraid to skip around your bedroom singing your revision notes if that is what works for you. There's no point in trying to revise in the same way as everyone else if it doesn't work for you.

4. **Highlight your notes, use different coloured pens, and make it interesting to look at:** When you experience inattention or hyperactivity, a repetitive and dreary task such as writing down revision notes can feel like dragging yourself through a swamp. You may find it easier to revise and study if you make it more stimulating by changing the

color of your pen when you feel bored, highlighting important aspects of the work, or moving onto revising in a different way. For example, if you have been taking notes on paper and you are struggling to continue, then move on to making notes on a whiteboard and take a photo of the notes when you are done.

5. **If you need a quick answer to a simple question, ask your phone's virtual assistant:** This can really help if you struggle with inattention to the point where you aren't able to read through countless articles to find the answer that you need. Your phone's virtual assistant may be able to give you the straightforward answer that you need.

6. **Turn assignment questions into mini worksheets:** An assignment about a particular topic may appear to only be asking one question, but is actually asking many. For example, if you are told to write an assignment about Tourette Syndrome, it isn't just asking you to write what the condition is - it may be asking you about potential management strategies, how it is represented in the media, the impact it can have on a person's life and many other aspects which are covered in the assignment topic. This is why some people find it helpful to create mini worksheets that split up a large assignment into smaller chunks. This allows people to ensure that they are covering every aspect of what they need to include, and not going on a tangent with unnecessary details.

7. **Do your best to start working earlier in the day if possible**: People tend to have higher levels of motivation when they start working on a project in the morning rather

than starting it in the afternoon. This may be because it makes a person feel accomplished and productive, and it may be that it tends to be sunny early in the morning and this helps people stay positive. As well as this, if a person doesn't start a task early in the day, they may just keep putting it off until the next day and never feel like it is the right time. Starting early can allow your mind to see that this is a priority.

8. **Don't be afraid to use practice papers /papers from previous years**: Exams can be daunting sometimes, but using practice papers or papers from previous years to revise can help you feel more comfortable with the layout of exam papers and can give you an idea of what to expect. Practice papers can also help you to plan your answers.

9. **Make sure that you eat enough and snack if you need to**: If you are hungry, then you are not going to be able to focus. Your brain needs nutrients, so you will find it much easier to think clearly if you have eaten enough.

10. **Use a metronome in the background to help you keep focused**: Some people find that focusing on the beat of a metronome in the background when studying helps them keep focused and stay on task. It prevents some people from daydreaming as there is a repetitive external noise which keeps bringing them back to the present. You can find metronome audio on online video platforms

11. **Revise in school**: In secondary school, people often

get a few weeks of "study leave" where they can go and revise at home. However, neurodivergent people often need clear boundaries between home life and school life, otherwise all of the stress associated with school can overtake home life. As well as this, people may be more easily distracted when trying to revise at home as all of their stuff is there - computers, tablets, games, etc. Due to this, some people find it easier not to go on study leave, and to continue going into school during this time to revise in the library. This allows the person to be in an environment where they are used to focusing on learning, and where they are less likely to be distracted. Doing "study leave" in school also makes it easier for a person to stick by their revision schedule as the ringing of the school bell will notify them when a certain amount of time has passed and the person may feel more pressure to focus on the task at hand if there are staff around, this can make it easier for some people to focus.

12. **Hyperfocus right before the exam:** Start revising early if you can and do your best to do it as much as you can, but as well as doing the typical level of revision, it can be helpful to hyperfocus on revision for around an hour before you go into the exam. People who are hyperactive and inattentive often work well under pressure, so this can help people take in some vital information right before the exam and can help you remember any facts and bits of information that you may have forgotten.

13. **Work with your tic cycles and take breaks when you need to:** There isn't much point in trying to revise on

a very bad tic day as you are unlikely to take much information in if you are constantly being disturbed by your tics, so try to focus more on revision sessions when your tics are milder.

14. **Try to find a clean and tidy environment to study in:** Some people find it easier to focus when they are in a clean and tidy environment, so it may be helpful to tidy up a bit before a study session if possible. Having a clean and tidy working space can help a person feel more motivated.

15. **Look after your mental health:** It can be easy to feel like every single moment of free time should be spent revising, but the reality is that this often isn't sustainable and can increase your stress levels, and therefore worsen your tics. Do take time to have breaks and perform activities that reduce your stress levels such as having a bath, listening to music, or watching a film every now and then. You can do this after a revision session as a little celebration to help you wind down.

Chapter Eleven

TOURETTE'S IN PUBLIC

Tourette's In Public

Sadly, a lot of people with Tourette Syndrome experience anxiety about going out in public due to fears around how their tics will be perceived. It can take time for an individual to develop the confidence to tic freely in public without anxiety, but it is possible.

If you are a parent of a Tourettic person reading this, it is vital **not** to encourage your child to hold their tics in when in public as this sends the message that their tics are shameful and should be hidden from the world. People need to be encouraged to tic freely whenever possible to reduce discomfort from the premonitory urges building up and to avoid an exacerbation of symptoms from suppression.

Some parents who are new to Tourette syndrome and have a child with swearing tics and socially inappropriate tics may wonder how on earth it is acceptable for them to be okay with their child doing those things in public. However, it is vital to remember that tics are involuntary neurological symptoms, just like seizures or tremors. There should not be any shame in a person experiencing a neurological symptom. Tics that involve swearing and socially inappropriate vocalizations are just like any other tic in the sense that they are not a reflection of the individual's personality and have no intention behind them and are, therefore, meaningless. If someone takes offense then it is never the fault of the Tourettic individual as they have a disability causing them to have neurologically misfired signals. A person should never be expected to harmfully suppress their symptoms just because other people are either uneducated or judgemental. It is, however, helpful if the Tourettic person is taught to explain their symptoms to others – some people find it helpful to carry a card around that explains TS so that they can quickly educate people on the condition.

There are only a few tics which can genuinely cause major problems in public. These include violent tics and sexual motor tics. These tics are less common, but can be socially debilitating. There are, however, ways to work around them, to allow someone to go out in public and function like anyone else. For example, if a person has a tic where they involuntarily hit out at others, they could just make sure that they maintain a safe distance away from people when they feel that tic coming so that they don't accidentally hit someone. Another example, if a person has a tic where they pull their trousers down, they could wear dungarees instead so that they can't be pulled down or they could wear a tight belt so that their tics are unlikely to be able to pull them down. It is vital not to punish a person for having these tics, because they are involuntary and the person doesn't want to be doing them.

Sadly, there are some situations where people don't really have an option not to suppress, for example, if there is any risk of serious physical harm to the Tourettic individual or those around them. If this is the case, people should try to get out of that situation as soon as possible so that they don't have to suppress for extended periods of time.

Some tips for dealing with tics in public for those with Tourette's are as follows:

- Never feel like you need to suppress your tics if there isn't any risk of serious physical harm. If someone has a problem with your tics, then it does not reflect you, it reflects them as they just don't understand.

- If you really don't feel comfortable ticcing in public due to anxiety or feeling that it is a situation that you can't tic in, then find something that makes your tics temporarily stop without having to consciously focus on holding them in and cause yourself immense discomfort. For example, some people may find that humming temporarily reduces their vocal tics and alleviates the urge to tic. Some people find that chewing gum helps to temporarily stop their tics and reduces the premonitory sensations. Do note though, that chewing gum shouldn't be used if there is a risk of you accidentally swallowing or inhaling the gum.

- In some circumstances, people may make rude comments about your tics. Try not to take offense at this as it is just a reflection of how ignorant and judgemental they are, not you. Try your best to learn how to stick up for yourself and challenge disability hate and discrimination.

- Some people find it helpful to wear a visual sign such as a hidden disability lanyard or a Tourette's awareness t-shirt to show people that they have a disability so that people will be understanding.

- Know that you never have to feel ashamed of your disability. The people who judge you are the ones who should be ashamed.

- People naturally stare when they are curious, or when they think someone seems interesting. Give them something to stare at!

- Sometimes you may find public places overwhelming due to the noise of people chatting and all of the bright lights, so don't feel afraid to wear sunglasses and/or ear defenders if you feel like they could help you.

You never need
to hide yourself
away from the
world due to
being Tourettic.

Chapter Twelve

EMPOWERMENT AND COMMUNITY

Meeting Others With Tics:

One of the main pieces of advice I would give to anyone starting off on their Tourette's journey would be to connect with other people with the condition, this can be done through online forums, social media groups and local support groups.

Meeting other people with the same condition allows you to embrace who you are. It will allow you to see that there are so many interesting, insightful, kind, caring and wonderful people with tics and it shows you that having this condition doesn't make you any less of a person. It shows you that people in the ticcing community have so many talents and that we shouldn't let our condition hide who we really are, we should instead use it to empower us.

Parents of people with Tourette's can also find it incredibly useful to go to support groups and connect with others on a similar journey. When the parents talk to adults who have the condition, it can give them an insight as to what it might be like for their child. The adults with TS know best what has helped them on their own journey, so they can share those experiences with the parents so that they can help their own child to thrive. Parents can talk with other parents to share the emotions they feel dealing with this condition, as Tourette's doesn't just affect the individual, it often has an impact on the whole family. Nobody can ever fully understand Tourette's or any other condition that causes tics unless they either have it themselves or have lived with and cared for someone who has it.

We are all in this together so meeting other people in the community allows you to feel understood on a deeper level. It gives you the ability to develop resilience, because you have the support of others who have endured the same symptoms and struggles. You can use their expertise, and you can see that they have gotten through this – so you can too.

It can be incredibly comforting to meet other people with the condition as you can share your experiences with self-doubt, anxiety, bullying, OCD and more in a completely non-judgemental environment. This gives you the ability to open up and not feel ashamed about your experiences as you have met others who relate to you. Sharing your experiences takes immense courage and you may inspire others to do the same.

Sometimes, when we go out in public, we may come face to face with ignorance, as people may not understand the condition and may wrongly assume that it's just 'bad behavior" when it's actually a highly misunderstood neurological condition. This misunderstanding may lead some people to become withdrawn and socially isolated but going to a support group can prevent these issues from surfacing in a variety of ways.

Firstly, many local Tourette syndrome support groups host fun activities that people of all ages can participate in, this provides a sense of community and entertainment so that you can socialize with people who understand and who are not going to judge as they have experienced similar struggles. They know exactly how it feels to be judged.

Secondly, you can talk to other ticcers to find out how they cope, and then you can implement these healthy coping methods for yourself.

Lastly, the connections and friendships you cultivate with others in the ticcing community can form very strong bonds as you are free to be your authentic self and you realize that it's okay to be vulnerable with these people as they want to help you. These are people to whom you can relate to on a deep level.

Going to a group and connecting with others who have the condition also gives you a great opportunity to discuss management strategies and gather information on how to liaise with schools and the workplace from people who have first-hand experience.

Everyone's experiences are different, as TS is a highly individualized condition with a diverse range of complex presentations and symptoms, but listening to other people's experiences can offer some much-needed reassurance and advice.

To find information on local support groups, you can contact a national or local Tourette syndrome organization, or inquire about local groups on a social media group. These online groups also give you the ability to post questions about the condition and share your experiences to receive 24/7 support from those who have been there. Community support is vital.

Just a word of warning about online support groups though, they can be a hotspot for arguments due to the wide range of experiences that different people have and the vast amount of people on the group hiding behind their profiles. In-person support groups tend to be a friendlier environment as people know each other and care about each other. Some online support groups are brilliant though, just be wary of the ones with a high level of censorship. Some groups will censor anything that goes against the admin's belief systems (for example, information on PANDAS/PANS, dietary tic triggers, histamine, alternative interventions, etc.) This can prevent people from finding out about things that may help them and change their lives for the better.

Some people do get very worried about whether going to a support group will make their tics worse. It is normal for tics to temporarily get worse when around others with tics. This exacerbation of tics can last a few days or weeks after leaving. It is also very common for people to pick up tics from other people as tics are highly suggestible. However, the pros of going to support groups usually outweigh the cons as people may learn management strategies that can be used to reduce the impact of their tics for life and may learn how to advocate for themselves which can alter the person's life path for the better.

Sometimes it feels like you are carrying a little bit of another person around with you if you pick up a tic from them. This can help us feel closer as a community and remember the unity of humanity.

The Importance Of Societal Acceptance:

I believe that as individuals with TS, we need to be valued for who we are and we need to feel empowered to speak up for ourselves. We shouldn't be asked to change, nobody should try to change us or try to fit us into a box of what society deems as acceptable, or try to stop us ticcing because of course, it's involuntary. (It is okay to use management strategies and medical interventions to help though, as that isn't "changing" us for the sake of fitting into a neurotypical box, but is there to help us.)

We should be given the support we need to fulfill our potential and to feel safe in an inclusive environment. It's vital because Tourette's can be very misunderstood, but the more awareness we raise, the more accepting society will be - therefore we will be more at ease in public. It will also be easier then to get access to appropriate support. It's important as when we are accepted, it does wonders for our self-esteem and confidence. If we aren't accepted or supported, we are likely to feel like an inconvenience. If that happens then it's heartbreaking as no one should have to feel ashamed for having TS or any other disability.

If people don't accept us and complain about our tics then it's vital for them to remember that our tics bother us much more than they bother other people. Although I do understand that some tics may seem disruptive - it is important to understand that we can't walk away from them when other people can and we also have to deal with all the co-occurring issues that come along.

We need to have our struggles acknowledged so that we can get support, but we also need to focus on our strengths because when we focus on our abilities – we feel encouraged to build upon them and work with them.

I believe that when we are accepted, we will feel more comfortable talking about our condition and we can then let our voices be heard. This would allow us to ask for support when we need it. We need to ask for help to be able to get it and with support, we can reach our true potential. This is why it's important to feel understood and be met with a non-judgemental stance from others when discussing our condition.

If you know someone with Tourette Syndrome then don't try to change them, but give them what they need to thrive and have the best quality of life possible. If they are struggling then you could support them in finding management strategies that can improve their quality of life. If the condition isn't bothering the individual or isn't having any significant impact on their lives then there are always ways to work around it with accommodations, modifications and being met with compassion and empathy. You don't have to try and change something that isn't causing any issues as I believe that any management strategy or treatment option is the individual's choice as we have freedom of autonomy (of course – as long as the person is in the right mental state to influence these things.) As long as we understand the pros and cons, we have a right to be involved in our care and management options. There are some circumstances though where parents may have to medicate a child even if the child doesn't fully understand it, these circumstances may be if a child is suffering but isn't in the right state of mind to consent or if the child is uncomfortable with change. In most circumstances however, the child should have a say in medication and if the tics aren't bothering the child then it may just help to embrace them rather than try to stop them. Repeatedly trying to stop the tics can harm an individual's self-esteem as they start to wonder "if the tics aren't bothering me, why are they bothering others? Am I an inconvenience?" Sometimes it isn't the tics themselves that cause problems, but it is the reactions we get from other people. If you are worried about the side effects of medications and the tics themselves are not causing significant problems, then educating the school or workplace and local community may be beneficial.

If you are the parent or carer of a child with Tourette Syndrome, please explain to them that any medication or intervention you give isn't to change who they are as a person as they are not broken, but is to help them manage and have a better quality of life. This open communication with the child can really build their trust and let them know that you are just doing your best to help them.

If we are in an accepting environment where we know that people understand our tics and aren't going to react negatively, then we become less anxious and therefore may tic less. Acceptance helps in many areas. If we don't know how people are going to react then our tics can get worse because we become hypervigilant, as if our tics are wondering if they are going to get a reaction. It's not us trying to get a reaction, but the tics will try their best to mortify us by trying to get people to react and notice them.

You may often worry when you're in new environments as you may wonder how people are going to react - will they be angry? Will they complain? Will they be discriminatory? When we are in a safe environment where people respond neutrally and do not react with offense, then we know that it's okay to let ourselves tic as we don't have to worry about accidentally upsetting others or being judged. Being in an accepting environment allows us to feel calm and focus on what we are working on, instead of being distracted by anxious thoughts such as "Are people judging me? Do they just think I'm disruptive?" It will also mean that people feel less of a need to suppress their tics.

Nobody should have to harmfully suppress symptoms to the detriment of their own well-being just to make people feel more at ease with their own ableism.

The question is, how do we create societal acceptance? The main avenue is through awareness and we can do this by being open about our experiences, which can be on social media or to friends, or by having the courage to ask for support when we need it. Another way is by correcting any misinformation out there - for example, people might make Tourette's jokes, not realizing how serious it really is, but we can respond in a constructive way by just reminding them that Tourette's and related conditions can actually be very serious and debilitating.

We have to tell people that the misconceptions and prejudices they have towards Tourettic people are incorrect and ultimately harmful to our community.

The Tourette's community is very diverse but people might make assumptions based on one person's experience when it's a very wide spectrum and they may also make assumptions based on stereotypes. When we feel supported, valued and accepted as we are, it helps us feel like we can embrace our authentic selves. We are not just defined by our Tourette's, but by who we are **with** our Tourette's. Please don't try to change us but do support us. If the person does need some sort of intervention to reduce the impact that the symptoms have on them, then you can assist them in finding something that helps - but please don't try to force anything unless seriously necessary.

When we are around people who understand, then we can go about our daily lives without fear. We won't feel the need to withdraw from social situations due to others' discomfort towards our differences and we can tic loud and proud whilst being open about our condition, and have the confidence to explain it to others.

Know that having Coprolalia never makes you a bad person. Coprolalia includes socially inappropriate, obscene and offensive tics. Some people worry that their coprolalia reflects some hidden part of them that could stem from subconscious judgments, but this is false.

Chapter Thirteen

TOURETTE'S AND MENTAL HEALTH

Factors That Harm The Mental Health Of Tourettic People

Tourette Syndrome is not a mental health condition. It is a neurological condition like Epilepsy or Parkinsons'. However, as mentioned before, mental health conditions such as OCD, Anxiety, and Depression often co-occur with Tourette Syndrome. Sometimes the Anxiety and Depression are caused by a person's neurological makeup, but sometimes they may be related to the stress of living with Tourette Syndrome.

There are many factors that can lead to poor mental health in Tourettic individuals:

- **Loneliness:** Sadly, some people get ostracized and teased by their peers, causing the Tourettic person to struggle to make friends. Some Tourettic people also feel anxious about leaving the house due to how other people react to their tics, preventing a person from attending social events.

- **Discrimination**: Many disabled people, including people with Tourette's, will experience some form of discrimination at one time or another. This could include being sent out of class for ticcing, being fired from a job due to judgements towards your symptoms, or being made to feel unwelcome in a public venue. Facing this kind of discrimination can leave a person feeling helpless, angry, victimized, and frustrated. It is important to remember though, that there are still so many nice people out there who wouldn't dream of being discriminatory and who will accept you as you are.

- **Not getting the appropriate accommodations:** If an individual doesn't get the accommodations that they need in order to function in school, university, or in the workplace - they will struggle a lot more. The individual may start feeling afraid of going into school for example, as they know they won't be able to cope without the extra support. This can lead to a lot of extra anxiety and can make a person feel helpless.

- **Medical gaslighting:** Some people have run-ins with doctors who do not understand the complexity of Tourette's. The doctors may give dangerous advice, refuse to give a diagnosis, refuse to refer to appropriate services or emotionally abuse the individual. This can leave a person feeling angry that they can't get the support that they need and frustrated that they aren't being listened to. It may also make the person feel afraid of seeing doctors in the future. The individual may feel helpless as they don't know where to turn for support. Do be aware, however, that if this has happened to you, there are still some great doctors out there who will be willing to help. It can just take time to find them.

- **Bullying:** Unfortunately, some people with TS get bullied by their peers. This can cause a person to feel isolated, afraid, and can lower self-esteem.

- **Being unable to live life in the same way as others:** Some people with TS may be unable to do certain activities, such as driving. This can make a person feel isolated and left behind if they see all their friends learning to drive, but they're unable to drive due to the severity of the tics.

What can be done to improve the mental health of Tourettic people?

Now that we've covered some of the factors that can harm the mental health of Tourettic people, it's time to focus on what can improve the mental health of people with the condition.

- **Find a support group:** Having the ability to attend Tourette's support groups can really help some people as it shows them that they aren't alone. It also allows the individual to get advice from other people with Tourette Syndrome, which can help the individual reduce the impact of the tics and navigate daily life with the condition.

- **Research the biochemical factors that contribute to poor mental health:** Poor mental health isn't always caused by something upsetting that has happened in a person's external environment. Our mental health comes from our brain, and physical issues in the body can impact the functioning of the brain, thus leading to poor mental health. Biological factors that can lead to severe psychiatric presentations include inflammation (which has been associated with Depression and Psychosis, even when a person does not have PANDAS/PANS) as well as vitamin and mineral deficiencies such as B12 deficiency. Food sensitivities and allergens can also play a role. It is important to make sure that a person doesn't have a physical disease that resembles a mental illness, such as Pyrrole disorder, Thyroid disorders, PANDAS/PANS, psychiatric manifestations of Lyme Disease and Bartonella, vitamin and mineral deficiencies, psychiatric manifestations of Coeliac disease, Neuropsychiatric MCAS, etc. If a person has physical issues underlying their poor mental health, then no amount of psychological therapy, antidepressants, or antipsychotics are going to get to the root of the problem. It is absolutely paramount that you take the time to research these factors using online research databases because the conventional medical system often doesn't delve deep enough to find a physical root for psychiatric symptoms so you will have to read the studies and scientific literature yourself. There are countless studies on these topics. Some people will seek the help of a functional medicine doctor to find the physical root of their psychiatric symptoms.

- **Ensure that the school or workplace provides accommodations:** People with Tourette Syndrome are intelligent and have a lot of potential. Accommodations and adjustments are often needed in school and in the workplace so that a person can access the tasks that they need to do without extra stress. Some students in the UK will need an Education, Health, and Care Plan in order to get the level of support that they need, but it is possible to receive a high level of support without an EHCP. Students in America may need an IEP or 504 plan.

- **Make sure that the person has fun in their life:** Living with Tourette syndrome and co-occurring conditions can be incredibly difficult. Having things to look forward to that distract the person from their struggles can help. Maybe try planning some fun weekend activities so that the individual has something entertaining to do. Encourage self-care activities such as having warm baths, doing yoga - or whatever makes the person feel calm.

- **Make social media a healthy place:** If your mental health is made worse by nasty comments from people who don't understand Tourette's, some social media platforms have a setting where you can ban certain comments containing specific words or phrases. Sometimes, it is more helpful to just not look at the comments. If anyone online harasses you about your condition or anything else, be sure to block them. If someone is making content that makes you feel shameful, anxious, or unhappy in some way - know that it is okay to unfollow them.

- **Find a doctor who truly understands Tourette's:** It can be frustrating if your doctor doesn't fully understand your condition. Make sure you find a doctor who listens to you, validates your experiences, and knows that you are the expert in your own condition. It is important that your doctor doesn't gaslight you or pressure you into doing therapies that you don't think will be helpful for you.

- **Know that there are therapy options other than CBT:** Cognitive Behavioral Therapy can help some people who are struggling with poor mental health by challenging irrational and unhelpful thoughts. However, CBT isn't helpful for everyone as some people find that it is invalidating and dismissive towards rational concerns. In these cases, other therapies such as counseling, art therapy, and Acceptance and Commitment Therapy may be more helpful.

- **Know that deep breathing techniques aren't for everyone:** Deep breathing techniques can be very calming for some people, but for people with Tourette Syndrome, breathing techniques may trigger breathing tics or compulsions associated with sensori-motor OCD.

- **Let the individual (or yourself if you are the one struggling) do what they need to do to soothe themselves:** Self-soothing looks different for different people. It may be that having a bath is the only thing that soothes one person, for another person, self-soothing may involve playing a repetitive video game to calm the mind. Let the individual take breaks throughout the day when going through a rough patch to focus on self-soothing activities like these. This can give people time to calm themselves at intervals throughout the day.

- **Ensure that the individual is getting adequate nutrition:** Nutritional Psychiatry is an up-and-coming type of mental health care that focuses on how nutrition is vital when it comes to maintaining good mental health. We need nutrients to create certain neurotransmitters. For example, Tryptophan, Vitamin B6 and Magnesium are all needed in order for the body to create Serotonin (often dubbed the "happy chemical.") As well as this, numerous studies have highlighted the impact of the gut microbiome when it comes to our mental health. Our diet can directly influence our microbiome so it is important to eat lots of prebiotic foods.

Common Feelings That People With Tourette's Go Through:

Self-doubt:

Those of us with Tourette syndrome may go through a phase of self-doubt. This is where we start to question ourselves and worry that we may be 'faking it' or 'not trying hard enough to stop'. Although we know inside that we can't control our symptoms as we would never put ourselves through this, we worry whether we may be 'subconsciously doing it for attention' but this is just our anxiety playing tricks on us, but sometimes we may genuinely start to believe it and feel guilty.

It's important to know that many people with Tourette's go through this phase so it isn't just you. It can help to talk to others with Tourette's online who have the same feelings.

Some people may worry that their Tourette's is actually psychological rather than neurological, but even if it was then it still wouldn't be your fault as nobody chooses to have any sort of condition, whether it is neurological or not. Sometimes we may feel the need to validate ourselves to prove to ourselves that we are not doing this on purpose, you may look back on your early childhood and say 'Well I went through that then so it can't be fake' or 'Well I have this symptom as well, so it's genuine'. I want you to know that you don't need to validate yourself as it isn't your fault, regardless of what your anxiety is telling you and regardless of what anyone else thinks.

You are not faking it, this is a common phase that many of us go through but it can be very distressing. You are not an inconvenience, you are not a burden, you are not doing this on purpose, you are not attention seeking and please don't ever feel that you need to suppress all the time as it only makes things worse.

Once this phase passes, the other side is beautiful as you start to accept who you are, embrace your condition and use your experiences to help others and be part of the wonderful Tourette's community. When you start to accept it and stop doubting yourself then you feel free as you no longer feel the need to suppress your tics or mask who you are.

You soon come to realize that this condition isn't your fault and that your tics and other symptoms are involuntary. You may then feel empowered to claim your Tourettic identity and accept who you are. You gain the confidence to be able to stick up for yourself when facing ignorance or discrimination. These self-doubt feelings are a form of intrusive thought, and feeling the need to validate yourself can be a compulsion. Just seeing the self-doubt intrusive thoughts as part of the experience of having TS and connecting to others in the TS community who also have these thoughts can make you feel that this is just a phase of the TS journey. This helps you ignore the thoughts so that they will eventually go away.

Missing The Tics:

Some people say that if they don't tic for a while due to a management strategy that they're using (something like medication or a diet change) then they may actually start to miss their tics. This may sound quite strange because when we have our tics they can cause distress and we might not want them; they bother us, they can hurt us, and they can be horrible to deal with. However, some people may actually miss their tics once they have reduced or gone away for a while because, in a sense some people feel like it's part of their identity, they're known for ticcing and it's just a part of them. So, if there is something that reduces that, the individual may feel like they've just lost part of themselves.

It can also make you worry whether you are still valid in the Tourette's community or not. The answer is yes you are still valid and you do still belong, even if you don't tic now or your tics are a lot milder than most people's, or if you don't tic as much as you used to. You are still valid, you are still welcome in the community, and you can still have friends in the community - no one's going to sideline you for that. You've still got the condition, you've still experienced the struggles associated with it and people should really be happy for you that you have found something that helps you. If they're not, then you have to question whether they are the best friends to be with in the first place.

You are also still welcome to talk about your experiences if your tics are milder of course. You still have the right to share your experience if you want to and talk about it. You don't have to endure severe symptoms all of the time to be an advocate. It's possible that you went through a hard time when you were younger and you feel much better now. Maybe you found something that really helps you and your tics are milder and you wonder whether you're still a good advocate for the community, and the answer is yes. People need to hear from advocates with your perspective as well.

The Mental Stress Associated With Tic Suppression:

Suppressing tics not only feels physically intolerable and makes it hard to focus on your surroundings, but it may also make you feel anxious, tense, and on edge. Tics need to come out at some point and can't all just be bottled up.

The problem is that for many people, not suppressing can also be stressful, as there may be fears about how people will react to the tics. This is why it's vital for people around the Tourettic individual to be educated on the condition, and for the ticcer to be educated on how to stick up for themselves and explain their condition to others in public.

Developing Self-Acceptance:

Learning to accept and embrace your Tourette's is a really important step to improving your quality of life.

Here are some tips to help you accept and embrace your Tourette's :

- Some people find it embarrassing to talk to family members, friends or teachers about their Tourette's. This is why it's important to get in touch with other people from the Tourette's community so that you can talk to people who have been through similar situations so they can give you support and advice. You can get in touch with other people with TS through local support groups and online support groups.

- If you are a family member of someone with Tourette's, please don't force the individual to talk about things if they feel uncomfortable, in time they might start to become more comfortable so just wait and let them know that you are there for them.

- You will start to accept yourself when you realize that there's nothing wrong with being different. You may realize that Tourette's can come with strengths, such as increased empathy from knowing what it feels like to struggle. This may allow you to help others more, and have more compassion towards yourself.

- Researching Tourette's for yourself can really help you

understand your condition and can eliminate any internal judgment you may have. Once you realize that your symptoms are involuntary, you start to care less about how other people react because you know that this isn't your fault and that if someone reacts negatively then you know that it is nothing to do with you. It just shows that that person needs some education and awareness of Tourette's.

- If you stop suppressing your tics as much as possible and learn to embrace being a ticcer, it can help you mentally and allow you to accept yourself as you authentically are - tics and all.

- Watch documentaries with other people with Tourette's in them so that you can have role models and people you can relate to, as this can make you feel deeply understood. It can show you that there are some incredible people with Tourette's out there who are happy, kind, successful and raising awareness.

- Some people find it easier to be open about their TS on social media than in person, once you put it on social media people will probably see it but then they will realize that having Tourette's doesn't change the fact that you are a great friend and funny person. People will realize that your Tourette's is just a little extra and if people don't accept it then they don't deserve the privilege of being your friend. Some people find it helpful to make friends with others in the Tourette's community and over time you will find a friendship group of people who understand and who are non-judgemental.

Unfortunately, the journey to embracing and accepting your Tourette's isn't usually very simple. It can take years to accept yourself, but when you do, it is definitely worth it. Meeting others with Tourette's and seeing how awesome other Ticcers are shows you that Tourette's can be one of your greatest assets. Go where you are accepted and ignore the people who don't understand because that it is just their own problem.

Accepting yourself can really help you mentally. You do not need the validation of others.

Know that if anyone judges you for your tics or makes a nasty comment, it is never a reflection of you. You cannot control your tics but most people can control how they respond.

Chapter Fourteen

TICS THROUGH THE SEASONS

Tourette's, Celebrations, & Religious Holidays

Celebrations such as religious holidays and birthdays can be incredibly exciting, the problem is that excitement can be a tic trigger for some people. Many families report having to "play down" any celebrations so that the individual with Tourette's doesn't experience an exacerbation in tics or OCD from excitement. This can be slightly disappointing to the individual, but is sometimes necessary in cases where a worsening of tics or OCD could be dangerous or cause immense distress.

There are however, factors other than excitement that can lead to tics getting worse around the time of celebrations and holidays. Some of the other factors which may cause tic exacerbations around these times are listed below:

1. **Sensory Overload:** Many people with Tourette Syndrome struggle with sensory processing issues. Sensory sensitivities can be a trigger for tics for some people. Holidays and celebrations bring more overwhelming sensory input into a person's life - repetitive songs, light displays with flashing lights, sparkly decorations, noisy shopping centers, etc. This can be incredibly overwhelming for someone with a highly sensitive nervous system.

2. **Dietary Changes:** As explained earlier in this book, some people find that certain foods make their tics worse.

Many people will have a different diet when it comes to the holiday season and celebrations. They may consume more sugary foods, chocolate, foods containing dyes, cheese, and more. These are possible trigger foods for some people, so sometimes the increase in tics seen can actually be caused by the changes to the individual's diet around this time. Some people find it helpful to see which foods have been consumed more often than usual when having a severe flareup of tics, because this helps them identify trigger foods so that they can be consumed less in the future and tasty alternatives can be found.

3. **Changes in routine and increased social interaction**: For individuals who are Autistic as well as Tourettic, changes in routine and increased social demands can cause intense stress and can therefore worsen tics.

Tips For Coping With Tic Flare-ups In The Holiday Or Celebration Season:

- Have a room in the home that does not contain any decorations so that a person is able to step away from the hustle and bustle and take a time out from the celebrations. This can prevent a person from becoming too overwhelmed.

- Let the person skip certain social events if they are not feeling up to it. Some people won't be able to cope with as much social interaction as neurotypical people as it may just increase their anxiety.

- Try to explain Tourette Syndrome to family members and friends whom you are celebrating with so that they know why the Tourettic individual is struggling and so that they know that it isn't a behavioral problem. You could print out some leaflets for them to read if it will help them understand.

- Be careful with diet changes. Offer food dye-free alternatives to the usual foods that people consume during the holiday season and observe how an individual's tics and other symptoms respond to increased consumption of cheese (dairy) and sugary foods. Reactions are usually delayed so tend to show up a few hours after consumption, this is because the type of food sensitivity that is associated with neurological symptoms is often fueled by immunoglobulin G which causes delayed reactions rather than immediate ones.

- If an individual's tics are triggered by flashing lights, then it would be best to avoid using these in your decorations and give the ticcer tinted lenses when out in public near light displays.

- Know that you do not need to do everything in the traditional way. Tourette Syndrome will mean that the whole family has to function differently, but that's okay. You do not have to celebrate in exactly the same way as everyone else.

Seasonal Tics: Tics can occur in context and can be observational, they are also very suggestible. Due to this, some people get a new set of tics during the holiday season that are relevant to that time of year. For example, around Halloween time, a person may start ticcing about pumpkins or trick or treating, and around Christmas they may start ticcing about Santa or elves. Seasonal tics are nothing to worry about, and can actually be quite entertaining and lighthearted for some people.

What if the tics get worse at specific times of the year such as during the summer or when a person returns to school?

If a person's tics get worse during a certain season, look at the pollen count during that time. The same as how some people find that food sensitivities exacerbate their tics, environmental allergens such as pollen sometimes can as well. People with Tourette Syndrome have higher rates of allergic diseases than the general population (Chang et al., 2011). Discomfort and inflammation triggered by allergies could potentially worsen tics. Pollen often triggers PANS flares as well as it triggers off the immune system.

If a person's tics get worse when returning to school after a holiday, this could be because of the stress of going back to school, changing their routine, and having to be around other people. It is also possible that it could be caused by the individual being exposed to so many people that their immune system gets inundated with germs from other people which could make tics worse if a person has undiagnosed PANDAS/PANS.

Chapter Fifteen

WHY ARE SYMPTOMS MORE PROMINENT IN CERTAIN ENVIRONMENTS AND NOT SO MUCH IN OTHERS?

Why can tics and other symptoms occur more in one environment and not so much in others?

Many family members of children with Tourette syndrome notice that the individual may display minimal symptoms in the school environment but once they reach the home setting their symptoms explode to the point of severe disability. This is almost like a 'Jekyll and Hyde' effect where there is a dramatic contrast between how the condition presents in different settings. Unfortunately, the misunderstanding as to why this phenomenon occurs may lead to parents being wrongly judged, blamed or left doubting their parenting skills from the assumptions made by medical professionals, school staff and extended family members. The symptoms often come out more in the home setting because it's our safe space where we know we won't be judged, not because there's anything wrong with the home environment or parenting. Neurological symptoms are NOT caused by bad parenting.

Another reason why someone may display more frequent and intense symptoms in a specific setting may be due to environmental tic triggers that are present. Many people find that tics and other neurological symptoms can be exacerbated by environmental allergens and sensory stimuli, these triggers can include (but are not limited to) air fresheners, dust, pollen, certain chemicals present on furniture, candles, cleaning products, mold, fluorescent lights, bright lights, flashing and flickering lights and more. When exposed to these triggers in certain environments, our tics can be set off and get worse very quickly.

We often have extremely sensitive nervous systems. Therefore, if tics occur more in certain environments such as in public settings, around certain triggers and when the individual hasn't been suppressing - then environmental factors could be something to look into.

Many people with Tourette's unfortunately knowingly or unknowingly suppress symptoms in the school environment or other public places, but any symptoms that are suppressed will always need to come out at some point as they accumulate over time and this can come out in extreme rebounds. It helps if people with Tourette's are encouraged to tic freely, so the safest space is often in the home environment. Parents may face misunderstanding from certain medical and support services. Sadly, some families have been sent to family counseling, sent to parenting classes, told that they need to discipline their child better, refused access to vital medical services, or have had symptoms dismissed and have been spoken to in a very condescending way when discussing a potential diagnosis. This can be incredibly stressful.

Rage attacks may also predominantly occur in only one environment, which is typically the home environment. This can also cause parents to be judged on their parenting skills, but you cannot discipline out a neurological condition. Rage comes out more at home as we know that we are safe there and are unlikely to be judged for a neurological symptom.

I would like every parent reading this to know that you know your child best and you see what they experience on a daily basis and the impact that it has on their lives and your own. Know that you are not alone and unfortunately, many parents do face this harsh and inaccurate judgment. Please know that you are trying your best as a parent and you shouldn't take advice from someone who doesn't understand the situation. Things do improve and over time you may receive the correct diagnosis and support. Trust yourself and know that things do work out and there will be people who understand. You are your child's best advocate, and they can learn from you how to be their own advocate, so keep seeking help from doctors and specialists who can understand the situation and don't stop until your child is receiving the most effective support that suits them - but also be sure not to automatically believe everything the doctors say (they can make harmful judgments.)

Chapter Sixteen

TOURETTE'S AND IDENTITY

The Impact Tourette's Has On A Person's Identity

Tourette Syndrome isn't all that a person is, but the impact that the condition has on the individual can impact how they see themselves, and the world.

Some people like to see Tourette's as a part of their identity and find that empowering. They may love getting involved in anything to do with TS awareness, such as wearing awareness merch and taking part in campaigns. This is because Tourette Syndrome can impact every area of an individual's life. In some ways, it can have a negative impact which makes us passionate about raising awareness and gives us a sense of compassion to want to help others who are also struggling. Some of the impact, however, may actually be positive. For example, it may increase a person's connection to a spiritual source as it gives them a sense of purpose in life - to raise awareness. It may even increase a person's confidence if they say to themselves "I've been through so much living with TS that I can get through anything". In this sense, the impact that Tourette Syndrome has on a person's identity can be positive.

It's also possible for a person to not see Tourette's as part of their identity and want to move as far away from the "label" as they can, this is also a valid way to feel. Though, being able to accept our differences can give us confidence and it isn't healthy just to see it as a "label."

A negative way that it can impact a person's identity is if they develop the idea that having Tourette's is a weakness, a lack of willpower, or something to hide. This will make a person judge themselves, have little confidence, and be disconnected from who they are as a whole.

The defining factor that determines if someone will see Tourette's as a positive part of their identity or a negative one is what messages have been sent to them throughout their journey. If the person has been told to suppress tics, has been pressured to "normalize" themselves out of shame, has been ignored when ticcing, or has been bullied a lot – then it will likely have a negative impact on their identity. However, if a person has been taught that it is okay to be unique, that it is not their fault if people react negatively to their tics, has been mentored by confident ticcers, and has been shown that Tourettic people can be successful – then it will likely have a positive impact on the way they see themselves and the relationship that they have with their condition.

Shame and low self-esteem are not symptoms of Tourette Syndrome, they are a consequence of not being accepted for who we are. For some, Tourette's can be something to embrace.

If a Tourettic individual is made aware of the strengths associated with having TS, it may help them feel more confident and accept themselves more. One strength is that some people with TS are highly energetic due to having ADHD tendencies, this can come in handy when it comes to sports. Some people with Tourette Syndrome are also very talented in a specific area such as music or art.

Many people find that focusing on a topic of interest can temporarily reduce tics, which can make someone better at their specific tic-reducing activity as they may spend a lot of time doing it as a coping mechanism.

Many people with Tourette's have a sensitive nervous system leading to sensory sensitivities and emotional overwhelm, but some people may feel like this allows them to be more in tune with and aware of the environment around them - making them more intuitive and empathetic.

Being in connection with others in the TS community can bring an amazing sense of unity, with the knowing that there are people on the other side of the planet going through the same thing and who would understand. It really reminds you that it is a "small world" so to speak.

Some people's tics are extremely quick and witty, the person's tics may reply to something in their environment without the person even needing to think. This quick humorous response from the tics can give someone a great sense of humor.

Many vocal tics are focused on syllables and specific sounds, for example, a tic may automatically come out with a specific number of syllables to satisfy the urge to tic, and the urge to tic may not be able to be satisfied unless the vocal tic contains a sharp sound such as "ca" or "ch". This can cause someone to be hyper-aware of the syllables and word sounds used in day-to-day life, which may translate into being a gift when trying to write poetry.

Many people with Tourette's have a lot of empathy, as living with a misunderstood condition is hard and these difficulties may make an individual know what it is like to struggle and therefore be more sensitive to others needs.

As well as potentially giving a person unique strengths, Tourette's may play a role in a person's religious or spiritual belief systems, life goals, friendships, interests, clothing choices, and more. Below is a list of each aspect of life that TS may unexpectedly impact, and how it can impact each area in that way.

Religious and spiritual belief systems: Having Tourette's can cause someone to question their pre-existing religious and spiritual beliefs as the struggle of living with the condition can make people wonder "why would God make someone suffer in this way?" This could lead someone to abandon their religion. Some people may also end up abandoning their religion if people keep telling them that their TS is a sign of possession as this is a false statement which can hinder a person from fully accepting themselves and getting the support that they need.

On the contrary, Tourette Syndrome may strengthen some people's religious or spiritual beliefs as they may find that seeking comfort in a higher power is helpful. People may also see their TS as a kind of spiritual experience, there to teach them important life lessons such as courage, resilience, and persistence. Some people may feel like they have Tourette Syndrome for a reason, so that they can educate others about the condition and be more understanding towards other people. This can allow someone to feel in tune with the universe and feel like the universe is working through them.

Life goals: Living with a disability such as Tourette Syndrome will allow a person to see what is truly important in life. It can show someone what really deserves their time and focus. The struggles that TS causes can give the individual the desire to help others. All of these things will impact a person's life goals. For example, if someone finds that dietary changes reduce their tics, they may aim to become a nutritional therapist or naturopath, if someone has experienced mental health struggles associated with TS, then they may have the goal to be a psychologist one day so that they can help other people.

Friendships: Having a misunderstood condition like Tourette Syndrome means that not everyone will be kind and understanding. This is very sad, however, it can allow ticcers to easily determine who is worth being friends with vs. who is not going to be good for them. This can allow them to become a good judge of character and can allow them to eventually find the right people to make friends with. Some people attend Tourette Syndrome support groups and camps, these events are a great opportunity to make friends with people in the community. Friendships formed within the community may last a lifetime and allow you / your loved one to learn management strategies and both give and receive support from others who understand. Making friends with the right people can change a person's entire life trajectory.

Sadly, it is possible that the individual will make friends with the wrong kinds of people, especially at a young age. Some people may try to take advantage of a person with TS and may try to be their friend solely for entertainment or to look "cool" by being friends with "the Tourettic kid". Thankfully, these fake friendships usually don't last long.

Interests: Having a disability may make someone interested in topics related to their experience such as neurology, medical science, disability advocacy, disability law, disability history, etc. These new-found interests can turn into expertise.

Clothing choices: This sounds like a strange one, but having TS may impact the clothes that a person wears. This is because sensory processing issues are very common in the Tourette's community. If a person is sensitive to the feeling of collars on shirts, this may trigger neck tics so people may stop wearing these shirts. If a person can't cope with wearing tight clothing, they may wear baggy clothes. This may influence a person's style which can alter how they see themselves and therefore their identity and "aesthetic". Our experiences in life can also influence our style and fashion sense in other ways as well, such as dressing in a grunge or gothic fashion to appear strong and to express how much we have been through. Many people have noticed that alternative fashion styles are common among Tourettic people. I personally feel that this is because we are so used to being stared and gawked at anyway, that we might as well express ourselves in the way we want as we will get stared at and treated differently anyway. It is freeing in a way.

These are just some examples of how Tourette Syndrome can impact many areas of a person's life and influence their identity. You will never be able to fully understand Tourette's by just reading a list of symptoms out of a textbook. You will need to understand how it feels, the impact it can have, how it becomes a kind of identity, and how it can influence every aspect of a person's life - but not always in a bad way.

Only you know what is best for your body. Only you know what you need to do to cope and manage tics. Do not let people convince you to stop listening to your body.

Chapter Seventeen

TOURETTE'S IN THE WORKPLACE

Tourette's In The Workplace

The world of work can be daunting for a person with Tourette Syndrome. You / your loved one may worry about being judged by coworkers, being fired for something that is uncontrollable or may worry about whether the tics will impact the work.

It is vital to know that many people with Tourette's are incredibly talented and intelligent, employers just need to give us a chance. There are some jobs that people with TS may find difficult, but this is dependent on the individual, different jobs will be right for different people. Some people have the impression that a Tourettic person will never be able to do a job that requires a high level of motor control such as being a surgeon or a lumberjack, but some people with TS find that their tics stop when focusing on something intensely or when doing something highly physical. Therefore, for some people, their condition may not even impact their career options in this way.

When working in an office or with other people, a person with TS may worry that they are distracting or annoying their co-workers. It is important to know though, that once the condition is explained to people then they are usually understanding and the tics can become background noise. Remote working is also an option for people who do not feel comfortable around others - or for the co-workers if they have a problem with a person with TS being in the workplace. Some people with Tourette Syndrome may not feel comfortable with the idea of working with members of the public, but again, once the condition is explained to people then it often isn't a problem. If the person really doesn't feel comfortable around other people (possibly due to anxiety or co-occurring Autism) then they could look into jobs where they can be more independent. This could be something where they can work from home.

Self-employment could be an option for some people who have the means to do it, though this can sometimes be risky as not all businesses will be a success. Some people may find self-employment helpful as they can work on their own schedule, which means that if they have a tic attack, then they can just take a break and come back to the work later without worrying. Self-employment may also give a person freedom to work on what they feel able to work on, on each given day. For example, if a person is having a really bad day with their OCD symptoms, they may feel that they can't focus on writing. They could then spend the day taking photos of products that they are selling or planning the design of social media marketing posts and may then go back to writing product descriptions when they are feeling a bit better.

Stress is something that commonly exacerbates tics, and this can be difficult in the workplace. Having a task set by someone else with a deadline may make a person feel so stressed that they tic too much to even work on the project. This is another reason why self-employment can be helpful, because there may be less pressure as the person is their own boss. If self-employment isn't an option and a person has this struggle, then they could be given flexible working hours where they can take a break whenever their tics or stress levels get too difficult to manage and then they could just make up the time later on when they are feeling better.

If an employer seems to have a problem with the person having Tourette Syndrome, then it is vital that they are educated on the condition and can recognise the strengths that the person has. It is illegal in the UK to fire someone or refuse to hire someone on the basis of their disability.

Job Recommendations For Those Who Don't Feel Comfortable Working In A Public Setting:

- A job where you can work from home / remote working.
- A job where there is the option of a night shift, as fewer people are around then.
- An office job where you get your own individual office or only have to share it with one or two other people.
- A delivery driver (if the person's tics don't stop them from being able to drive.)
- An author - we live in a day in age where it is possible to self-publish books for free.
- Graphic designer - this is a job that doesn't require much social interaction.
- Computer Programmer.

To make it clear, I do not advocate for Tourettic individuals to work independently or to avoid the public, these recommendations are just for people who genuinely don't feel comfortable working with others due to anxiety.

We should never have to hide away from the world.

Possible Workplace Accommodations For Tourettic Individuals: (A guide for employers)

- Ensure that colleagues are informed about the individual's condition if the individual wants that information shared.

- Give the individual permission to take breaks as needed. The tics can change in severity and frequency from one minute to the next. The Tourettic individual may suddenly have a bad episode of tics where they are unable to continue the task at hand. People will often need to take a break to help their tics decrease again.

- Tasks that are interesting and engaging may reduce a person's tics as a lot of people find that their tics reduce when they are working on something that takes a lot of their focus. An accommodation could be delegating engaging activities to the Tourettic individual.

- Offer remote or hybrid working. Some people may have tic episodes or flares of co-occurring conditions so severe that they struggle to leave the house. Offering remote and hybrid options for Tourettic employees can allow the individual to work in a way that works for them. It must be the individual's choice, however – you cannot force them into remote working as this could be seen as discrimination.

- Many Tourettic people have sensory processing issues that can make them sensitive to noise and lights. Sensory overload may exacerbate tics for some people. Allowing the individual to wear headphones and/or sunglasses can be helpful.

- Allow the individual space to have a quiet working area. Being in a quiet environment may reduce the tics and limit distractions (many Touretters also have ADHD.)

- If possible, and if the individual has the ability to prioritize tasks - it can be helpful to give the individual a list of tasks that need to be done, and they can choose which task to do depending on how they feel on a given day.

- Encourage the use of assistive technologies when needed. Text-to-speech software may be helpful for individuals who struggle to read due to eye-rolling tics, blinking tics, or co-occurring struggles.

- If the individual cannot drive and struggles with being around a lot of people - consider adjusting their working hours so that they can use public transport to and from work at a quieter time.

- Seeing as many people with Tourette Syndrome also have traits of ADHD, provide written instructions instead of just verbal instructions as the individual may not be able to remember and retain verbal instructions.

You are never an inconvenience in any way.

Chapter Eighteen

"MILD" VS SEVERE CASES

"Mild" vs Severe Cases – The Considerations

Tourette Syndrome is a spectrum condition, this means that it is a condition which affects everyone in a different way and to a different extent. Saying that a condition is a spectrum condition does not mean it's a form of Autism – Tourette's is not a form of Autism, there are different spectrums. Tourette's falls on the tic disorder spectrum.

People who are labeled as having "mild" Tourette's face issues just like those with more severe and noticeable cases, however, people with more subtle forms of the condition are often ignored and invalidated.

As well as this, people with more severe presentations of the condition are often ignored, stigmatized, and ostracized within our own community.

Comments on "mild" Tourette's:

Just because a person's tics are classed as "mild" and are subtle, doesn't mean that the impact the tics have on the individual is mild.

Tics are often classed as mild if they are less noticeable to outsiders and if they don't involve more than one muscle group or full words.

Examples of "mild" tics:

- hard blinking
- eye rolling
- throat clearing
- neck stretching
- toe clenching

Despite these tics being labeled as "mild" they can still have a significant impact on the individual who is experiencing them. For example, excessive blinking and eye-rolling tics can impact a person's ability to drive and/or read, repetitive throat-clearing tics can cause awful throat pain, and toe-clenching tics can trigger excruciating foot cramps.

People with less noticeable tics are often invalidated because people will say "At least you don't have a more complex tic" and this can make the person feel like their struggles are ignored.

As well as this, having subtle tics doesn't mean that the individual doesn't need a high level of support. Even less complex tics can cause major struggles. As I said already, eye rolling and blinking tics may require a person to need help reading and they may need transport support due to being unable to drive due to not seeing properly.

Tic severity isn't an indication of the severity of the co-occurring conditions. Even if a person doesn't feel like their tics impact them at all - the same doesn't necessarily go for co-occurring conditions. These co-occurring conditions such as OCD and ADHD can impact an individual more than the tics themselves. These other struggles may be hidden and ignored as doctors and family members may only focus on tic severity and assume the person doesn't need much support if their tics are "milder."

You cannot tell how much support a person needs just by looking at them, and you don't know how much a person's condition really impacts them unless you ask them. Just because a person's tics seem "mild" - it doesn't necessarily mean that things are easy for them to deal with.

Comments on how people with more severe presentations of the condition are ignored and ostracized by our own community:

Sadly, people with more extreme and noticeable presentations of the condition tend to be ostracized from the greater Tourette Syndrome community. I have known people get banned from Tourette's groups all over the world for having tics that are "too severe" or which "involve swearing." It is awful that even our own community doesn't know how to support those with more complex presentations of the condition. Do not worry about going to support groups if you have severe tics though as most groups aren't like this - it's only been an issue in a minority of groups that don't have the services for those with more complex cases.

Some studies on interventions to help those with Tourette's leave out those with more severe tics - likely with good intention as they don't want to accidentally make a person's condition worse than it already is. However, if people with more severe presentations aren't included in studies then it can be problematic as results will then only be based on those with less complex forms of the condition, meaning that the results shouldn't be able to be generalized to everyone with TS. Sadly, I have seen the results of these kinds of studies being used to gaslight those with more complex and extreme forms of the condition for experiencing a certain trait that those with less complex forms of the condition don't have or for not responding to an intervention that those with "milder" tics find helpful.

People should never try to use study results to gaslight a person or disbelieve their personal experience. Studies can easily be manipulated and people with more complex forms are often turned away and told that they don't fit the exact criteria to take part in the study. As well as this, just because the majority of people with a condition respond well to something, doesn't mean that everyone will. Just because most people don't experience a certain trait, doesn't mean that no one does - so study results generalized to the majority shouldn't be used to dismiss everyone else's experiences.

Some people in the Tourette's community will repeatedly point out that swearing tics are rare and that they don't have them, as if they're trying to distance themselves from those who do have swearing tics. Swearing tics are just the same as any other tic, they are involuntary and have no meaning behind them. When others in the TS community constantly try to make out that the swearing tic is incredibly rare, it just makes this type of tic more stigmatized.

Some people in the Tourette's community also seem to get offended when people talk about rage attacks, which are a symptom of TS as Tourette's is much more than just tics. People get offended and angry as they "don't want to be associated with people who have rage attacks" even though the rages are an involuntary symptom that doesn't reflect an individual's personality - just like the tics. It is important to speak about rage attacks so that people who experience them don't get blamed, shamed, and emotionally abused for a symptom that is just as (if not more so) uncontrollable than the tics.

Content creators with milder / more subtle forms of the condition have been known to spread misinformation such as saying "contextual tics don't exist" or that "people with severe tics can't be happy and laughing whilst ticcing." Both of these statements are false and only serve to increase the judgment that those with more extreme tics face on a daily basis. I've also seen content creators with more subtle forms of the condition make fun of those with more outwardly noticeable and extreme forms, because they assume that these people must be faking when they're actually not - some people do just have very extreme and complex tics.

If we can't even accept others with the same condition as us, how on earth can we expect the general public to understand Tourette's?

We need to do better. We need to include people regardless of how their condition presents. We need to stop gaslighting those with more complex tics, we need to stop leaving them out of studies, and we need to stop ostracizing them from our own community.

You will probably experience self-doubt, there may be a little voice in your head telling you that you're "faking it", but you are not, many people with tics have this and if you are questioning whether you are faking it I can guarantee you are not.

Chapter Nineteen
ADVOCACY

Advocacy & Activism

Some Tourettic people decide to go into disability advocacy and activism so that they can raise awareness and use their experiences to help others in the community. Not only does this help the general public understand the condition, but sometimes it can help the Tourettic person grow in confidence and learn how to explain their condition to others.

Some people like to join charity groups to be an ambassador for a charity, and some people prefer to do independent activism. Activism as part of a charity group can allow someone to have training on how to be an activist, and can open up some opportunities to make it easier to have a public platform to use to raise awareness. Independent activism has its benefits too, as it can give you more freedom to talk about your experiences and not have to feel restricted by any rules.

Advocacy and activism can be done in many ways. A person can raise awareness by creating content on various social media platforms, or they can raise awareness at in-person events by doing talks or presentations in their local community. Regardless of how someone chooses to raise awareness, it is all valuable and appreciated; it can make a huge difference.

There are some potential negatives of advocacy, however, such as the accidental spread of misinformation, so it can be helpful for advocates to read studies, articles, and books about Tourette's and related conditions if they are talking about more than just their personal experiences.

Some people do struggle mentally from the stress of advocacy, for reasons such as the following:

- Some people may feel frustrated that they cannot get everyone to understand. Some people will hear information on the condition and just choose to ignore it. It is important to accept that your advocacy won't reach everyone, but for those who do listen, it can change their life.

- Some people may receive hate comments if they raise awareness through social media. These can be extremely hard to deal with and may make a person doubt themselves. If this is a problem, then a person can turn off commenting on their posts or just choose not to read the comments that they receive.

- Some people may become exhausted feeling like they are constantly cleaning up the mess caused by the media's representation of Tourette's and by doctors who work using outdated information. It is important to remember that it is not your responsibility to solve everyone's problems. You just do what you can, and whatever you put out there is adding something to the world that wasn't there before. You do not have to correct every single bit of misinformation or post every single time there is an issue in the disability community. Just follow your passion. What you can do is enough.

It is important to protect yourself online as a Tourettic person. Sadly, many people do receive hate comments surrounding their disability, which can harm the person's mental health.

Below are some ideas on how to protect yourself online as a person with TS:

- Some social media apps allow you to block comments containing certain words or phrases. Use this to your advantage to automatically have hateful and fakeclaiming comments blocked.

- If you find that social media is stressing you – take a break. It can be stressful to constantly hear about the struggles that others in the community are facing, so take a break from social media whenever you need to.

- Block anyone who harasses you with hateful comments or fake claims.

- Don't share the names of specific hospitals you go to or doctors you see. You can say general terms like "neurologist" and "psychiatrist" as long as you don't use your specific doctor's name.

- Oftentimes, it's best not to read comments... people who are happy with the post will usually just like it, it's often mainly those with something mean to say that feel the need to make themselves heard in the comments. The majority of people are kind and understanding, but those who are cruel just seem the loudest as they always try to make sure they're heard by leaving comments.

Fundraising:

Some people are so passionate about supporting others in the community that they decide to fundraise for a charity. It is incredibly important to research the pros and cons of each charity before donating to them, as you need to ensure that they center the voices of Tourettic people and that the money goes towards campaigns that help those in the community. Please be aware this does not refer to any specific charity and certainly not any I am affiliated with – you just have to make sure the charity you're supporting aligns with your views and aims.

Fundraising Ideas:

- Do a sponsored run.
- Stay awake for 24 hours and have people sponsor you to do that.
- Sell jewelery that you make.
- Encourage your school or workplace to do a non-uniform or silly jumper day where everyone brings in some money to donate.
- Ask family members to donate money to a charity on your birthday.

Nobody should ever have to feel ashamed of having Tourette syndrome or tics. The people who bully, ridicule and discriminate against those with tics should be ashamed of their behavior. Often it is better to have Tourette's / tics than to be a person who bullies and ridicules those who have differences.

Chapter Twenty

FINAL THOUGHTS

Final Thoughts

I really hope that this book has been helpful in allowing you to understand yourself or your child a little bit better. Tourette Syndrome can be a very difficult condition to live with, but the more we learn about the condition, the easier it can become to manage.

Tourette Syndrome can be something to be embraced, something which makes us into a better version of ourselves, allows us to embrace being unique, and become passionate about raising awareness. Being unique is a beautiful thing, no one can change the world unless they bring something different to the world.

I want to thank all of the older adults in the Tourette's community for being role models to me. I want to thank my parents for always doing research and advocating for me, and I also want to thank the teachers I had in school and college who accepted me as I was and supported me.

Disclaimer: None of the information in this book should be seen or taken as medical or legal advice - it is all based on my own lived experience and what I have learnt throughout my own journey. It should be used for educational purposes only to help Tourettic people understand themselves more, and to help their families understand as well. For medical advice - see a qualified neurologist, neuropsychiatrist, psychiatrist, psychologist, or other medical professional with expertise in Tourette Syndrome and related conditions. Information on management strategies and treatments should not be seen as recommendations.

Recommended Reading:

The following are some other books that I would personally recommend, relating to Tourette Syndrome and co-occurring conditions.

Tourette's Books:

- **Hi I'm Adam: A Child's Book about Tourette Syndrome** by Adam Buehrens
- **My Non-identical Twin** by Evie Meg
- **Natural Treatment for Tics and Tourette's** by Sheila Rogers Demare
- **Stop Your Tics By Learning What Triggers Them** by Sheila Rogers Demare
- **The Man Who Mistook His Wife For A Hat** by Oliver Sacks (Tourette's is mentioned in a couple of chapters)
- **Tics and Tourette Syndrome: A Handbook for Parents and Professionals** by Uttom Chowdhury

OCD books:

- **Obsessive Compulsive Disorder: A Practical Guide** by Martin Dunitz
- **Problems In The Behavioral Sciences - Theoretical Approaches To Obsessive Compulsive Disorder** by Ian Jakes
- **What to Do When Your Brain Gets Stuck: A Kid's Guide to Overcoming OCD** by Dawn Huebner and Bonnie Matthews

Recommended Reading:

PANDAS/PANS Books:

- **Brain Under Attack: A Resource for Parents and Caregivers of Children with PANS, PANDAS, and Autoimmune Encephalitis** by Beth Lambert and Maria Rickert Hong
- **Childhood Interrupted: The Complete Guide to PANDAS and PANS** by Beth Alison Maloney
- **Saving Sammy: A Mother's Fight to Cure Her Son's OCD** by Beth Alison Maloney
- **Shadow Syndromes: Shining a Light on PANS and Other Inflammation-Based Illnesses Plaguing Today's Youth** by Anymom
-

ADHD Books:

- **Dirty Laundry: Why adults with ADHD are so ashamed and what we can do to help** by Richard Pink and Roxanne Emery
- **How Not to Fit In: An Unapologetic Guide to Navigating Autism and ADHD** by Jess Joy and Charlotte Mia
- **How to ADHD: An Insider's Guide to Working with Your Brain (Not Against It)** by Jessica McCabe
- **It's Never Just ADHD: Finding the Child Behind the Label** by Sandra Coral
- **UNMASKED: The Ultimate Guide to ADHD, Autism and Neurodivergence** by Ellie Middleton

References:

1 . Belluscio, B.A., Jin, L., Watters, V., Lee, T.H. and Hallett, M. (2011). *Sensory Sensitivity To External Stimuli In Tourette Syndrome Patients.* Movement Disorders, 26(14), pp.2538–2543. doi:https://doi.org/10.1002/mds.23977.

2. Berk, M., Williams, L.J., Jacka, F.N., O'Neil, A., Pasco, J.A., Moylan, S., Allen, N.B., Stuart, A.L., Hayley, A.C., Byrne, M.L. and Maes, M. (2013). *So Depression Is an Inflammatory Disease, but Where Does the Inflammation Come from?* BMC Medicine, [online] 11(1). doi:https://doi.org/10.1186/1741-7015-11-200.

3. Bitsko, R.H., Danielson, M.L., Leeb, R.T., Bergland, B., Fuoco, M.J., Ghandour, R.M. and Lewin, A.B. (2020). *Indicators of Social Competence and Social Participation Among US Children With Tourette Syndrome.* Journal of Child Neurology, 35(9), pp.612–620. doi:https://doi.org/10.1177/0883073820924257.

4. Cavanna, A.E., Robertson, M.M. and Critchley, H.D. (2007). *Schizotypal Personality Traits In Gilles De La Tourette Syndrome.* Acta Neurologica Scandinavica, 116(6), pp.385–391. doi:https://doi.org/10.1111/j.1600-0404.2007.00879.x.

5. Chang, Y.T. et al (2011). **Correlation of Tourette Syndrome and Allergic Disease: Nationwide Population-based Case-control Study.** Journal of developmental and behavioral pediatrics: JDBP, [online] 32(2), pp.98–102.
doi:https://doi.org/10.1097/DBP.0b013e318208f561.

6.Cox, J.H. and Cavanna, A.E. (2015). *Irritability Symptoms In Gilles De La Tourette Syndrome.* The Journal of Neuropsychiatry and Clinical Neurosciences, 27(1), pp.42–47.
doi:https://doi.org/10.1176/appi.neuropsych.13060143.

7. Darrow, S.M. et al (2017). *Autism Spectrum Symptoms In A Tourette's Disorder Sample.* Journal of the American Academy of Child & Adolescent Psychiatry, [online] 56(7), pp.610–617.e1.
doi:https://doi.org/10.1016/j.jaac.2017.05.002.

8. Dölp, A., Schneider-Momm, K., Heiser, P., Clement, C., Rauh, R., Clement, H.-W., Schulz, E. and Fleischhaker, C. (2020). **Oligoantigenic Diet Improves Children's ADHD Rating Scale Scores Reliably In Added Video-Rating.** Frontiers in Psychiatry, 11.
doi:https://doi.org/10.3389/fpsyt.2020.00730.

9. Eddy, C.M., Mitchell, I.J., Beck, S.R., Cavanna, A.E. and Rickards, H. (2011). *Social Reasoning In Tourette Syndrome.* Cognitive Neuropsychiatry, 16(4), pp.326–347.
doi:https://doi.org/10.1080/13546805.2010.538213.

10. Egger, J., Graham, P.J., Carter, C.M., Gumley, D. and Soothill, J.F. (1985). **Controlled Trial Of Oligoantigenic Treatment In The Hyperkinetic Syndrome.** The Lancet, 325(8428), pp.540-545. doi:https://doi.org/10.1016/s0140-6736(85)91206-1.

11. Gabbay, V., Coffey, B.J., Guttman, L.E., Gottlieb, L., Katz, Y., Babb, J.S., Hamamoto, M.M. and Gonzalez, C.J. (2009). *A Cytokine Study In Children And Adolescents With Tourette's Disorder.* Progress in Neuro-psychopharmacology & Biological Psychiatry, 33(6), pp.967-971. doi:https://doi.org/10.1016/j.pnpbp.2009.05.001.

12. García-López, R., Romero-González, J., Perea-Milla, E., Ruiz-García, C., Rivas-Ruiz, F. and de Las Mulas Béjar, M. (2008). *An Open Study Evaluating the Efficacy and Security of Magnesium and Vitamin B(6) As A Treatment of Tourette Syndrome In Children.* Medicina Clinica, [online] 131(18), pp.689-691. doi:https://doi.org/10.1157/13129113.

13. Garris, J. and Quigg, M. (2021). *The Female Tourette Patient: Sex Differences In Tourette Disorder.* Neuroscience & Biobehavioral Reviews, 129, pp.261-268. doi:https://doi.org/10.1016/j.neubiorev.2021.08.001.

14. Gerrard, J.W., Richardson, J.S. and Donat, J. (1994). **Neuropharmacological Evaluation Of Movement Disorders That Are Adverse Reactions To Specific Foods.** The International Journal of Neuroscience, [online] 76(1–2), pp.61–69. doi:https://doi.org/10.3109/00207459408985992.

15. Kozlowska, K., Chung, J., Cruickshank, B., McLean, L., Scher, S., Dale, R.C., Mohammad, S.S., Singh-Grewal, D., Prabhuswamy, M.Y. and Patrick, E. (2018). **Blood CRP Levels Are Elevated In Children And Adolescents With Functional Neurological Symptom Disorder.** European Child & Adolescent Psychiatry, 28(4), pp.491–504. doi:https://doi.org/10.1007/s00787-018-1212-2.

16. Kwak, C., Vuong, K.D. and Jankovic, J. (2003). **Migraine Headache In Patients With Tourette Syndrome.** Archives of Neurology, 60(11), p.1595. doi:https://doi.org/10.1001/archneur.60.11.1595.

17. Ludlow, A.K. and Rogers, S.L. (2017). ***Understanding the Impact Of Diet and Nutrition On Symptoms Of Tourette Syndrome: A Scoping Review.*** Journal of Child Health Care, 22(1), pp.68–83. doi:https://doi.org/10.1177/1367493517748373.

18. Martino, D., Zis, P. and Buttiglione, M. (2015). ***The Role Of Immune Mechanisms In Tourette Syndrome.*** Brain Research, [online] 1617, pp.126–143. doi:https://doi.org/10.1016/j.brainres.2014.04.027.

19. Müller-Vahl, K.R., Buddensiek, N., Geomelas, M. and Emrich, H.M. (2008). **The Influence Of Different Food And Drink On Tics In Tourette Syndrome.** Acta Paediatrica (Oslo, Norway: 1992), [online] 97(4), pp.442-446. doi:https://doi.org/10.1111/j.1651-2227.2008.00675.x.

20. Rodrigo, L., Álvarez, N., Fernández-Bustillo, E., Salas-Puig, J., Huerta, M. and Hernández-Lahoz, C. (2018). **Efficacy Of A Gluten-Free Diet In The Gilles De La Tourette Syndrome: A Pilot Study.** Nutrients, 10(5), p.573. doi:https://doi.org/10.3390/nu10050573.

21. Trillini, M.O. and Müller-Vahl, K.R. (2015). **Patients With Gilles De La Tourette Syndrome Have Widespread Personality Differences.** Psychiatry Research, 228(3), pp.765-773.
doi:https://doi.org/10.1016/j.psychres.2015.04.043.

22. van der Feltz-Cornelis, C., Brabyn, S., Ratcliff, J., Varley, D., Allgar, V., Gilbody, S., Clarke, C. and Lagos, D. (2021). ***Assessment Of Cytokines, MicroRNA And Patient-related Outcome Measures in Functional Neurological Disorder (CD/FND): The CANDO Clinical Feasibility Study.*** Brain, Behavior, & Immunity - Health, 13, p.100228. doi:https://doi.org/10.1016/j.bbih.2021.100228.

Your condition doesn't define you.

You define you.